Praise for *Life in the Balance*

"An inspiring story from a brave and spirited woman. Dr. Marla reminds us that life is tenuous and precious and needs to be treasured." —Lloyd Robertson, Chief Anchor and Senior Editor, *CTV News*

"A stunning tale, powerfully told. . . . Anybody contending with cancer will feel less lonely with [Dr. Marla's] words next to them. But the people who will most need to read this book are the galaxy of friends, family, co-workers and doctors who surround all cancer patients." —Andy Barrie, CBC Radio

"In *Life in the Balance*, Dr. Marla is visited by almost unspeakable pain and heartache. The strength of her character shines through on every page." —Vicki Gabereau

"Informative, touching and even funny. A great addition to the breast cancer literature." —Dr. Susan Love, MD, President and Medical Director of the Dr. Susan Love Research Foundation and author of *Dr. Susan Love's Breast Book*

"Marla's book is raw and painful and honest. She . . . tells a remarkable personal story with the ring of truth. Marla couldn't be stronger or more driven, but cancer has made her more mindful. She learns and teaches the hard lessons very well." —Valerie Pringle

"Dr. Shapiro is able to connect to the reader as she connects to her patients. Her own personal struggles with health demonstrate to us that one's personal strength is key to recovery. I consider her one of the great women of our time." —Art Smith, Personal Chef to Oprah Winfrey and author of *Back to the Table* and *Kitchen Life*

"An unsentimental insight into survival and resilience. Marla Shapiro generously shares some pretty tough life lessons from her defiant and single-minded battle with breast cancer." —Hana Gartner

"Marla Shapiro's incredible story of courage and determination will touch the hearts of all who read this powerful book. It is truly inspiring." —Bonnie Stern

LIFE IN THE BALANCE

LIFE IN THE BALANCE

MY JOURNEY WITH BREAST CANCER

DR. MARLA SHAPIRO

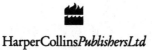

HarperCollins*PublishersLtd*

Published by HarperCollins
Publishers Ltd

First published in hardcover by HarperCollins Publishers Ltd: 2006
This trade paperback edition: 2007

Articles from *The Globe and Mail* (Oct. 26, 2004: "In a healthy balancing act, one ball is easier to juggle than two," and Mar. 15, 2005: "Shelve the blame game: Stress doesn't cause breast cancer") are reproduced courtesy of *The Globe and Mail.*

Excerpts adapted from *Not Dead Yet* and *Cancer Is a Word, Not a Sentence,* by Dr. Robert Buckman, are used by kind permission of the author.

The recipes found on pages 311–18 are © Bonnie Stern Cooking Schools Ltd., and are reprinted with permission.

The training regimen found on pages 319–31 are © Dr. Stacy Irvine and are reprinted with permission.

HarperCollins books may be purchased for educational, business, or sales promotional use through our Special Markets Department.

HarperCollins Publishers Ltd
2 Bloor Street East, 20th Floor
Toronto, Ontario, Canada
M4W 1A8

www.harpercollins.ca

Library and Archives Canada Cataloguing in Publication

Shapiro, Marla
Life in the balance : my journey with breast cancer / Marla Shapiro.

Includes index.
ISBN-13: 978-0-00-224384-1   ISBN-10: 0-00-224384-9

1. Shapiro, Marla–Health. 2. Breast–Cancer–Patients–Canada–Biography.
3. Physicians–Canada–Biography. 4. Television journalists–Canada–Biography. I. Title.

RC280.B8S49 2006   362.196'994490092   C2006-903956-9

Printed and bound in the United States

HC 9 8 7 6 5 4 3 2 1

Design by Sharon Kish
Set in ITC New Baskerville

For more information about cancer and the Canadian Cancer Society, please visit *www.cancer.ca* or call 1-888-939-3333.

To Bobby, Jenna, Amanda and Matt—my reasons for being

Contents

PART THREE

THE VIEW FROM HERE

PART FOUR

THE JURY SPEAKS

Foreword

In *Life in the Balance: My Journey with Breast Cancer*, Dr. Marla Shapiro sensitively and perceptively describes the double pressures (and more!) of being a breast cancer patient as well as being a physician—and Canada's most well-known and much admired doctor at that.

In honest and accessible terms, she explains the emotional impact of the diagnosis, the effect it has on her, her family, her career and her sense of balance; in addition she portrays the deep urge to know the best route to follow at every medical crossroads and to be in control of her own treatment. As her book well shows, there are many difficulties entailed in that double role.

Perhaps the most significant message from this book is that there may not be a single, obvious and compelling "One Right Answer" to every clinical problem. In many cases—as illustrated well by Dr. Marla's conversations with Dr. Susan Love—there may be several appropriate and acceptable answers, and the path that any person chooses may also depend on how that individual assesses the risks, the potential benefits, the side-effects, the impact of the treatment on the patient and the family and—in its widest and most accurate meaning—the quality of life.

A large number of my patients with breast cancer have said how Dr. Marla's example inspires them, and makes them feel better able to cope and understand their situation. This book will greatly add to that effect and is a welcome portrayal of the difficulties, the obstacles, the setbacks and the frustrations as well as the victories, the gains and (unexpectedly) the benefits of potentially serious illness.

—Dr. Robert Buckman, Medical Oncologist, Princess Margaret Hospital, and Professor, University of Toronto

PART ONE

OUTSIDE, LOOKING IN

ONE

Who I was

I have never been a superstitious person. After all, I am a doctor and have been trained to believe in science and evidence, to make a diagnosis and move forward with the best steps towards management—trained to take control. But it is true that as a doctor there have been times when I was overwhelmed by the inability to take control, times when I have been powerless to intervene and could only stand by, hoping to make things easier, if not better. So it was ironic that on Friday the 13th—August 13, 2004, to be exact—I was diagnosed with breast cancer.

That diagnosis and everything that followed came to define my life for a time and would ultimately change me forever. It marked an invisible boundary, a before and after, by which everything in my life—and in the lives of my husband and children—would be measured. As I stood in the hallway of the mammography suites, listening to the words "suspicious for breast cancer," a feeling of powerlessness came over me. I knew I was taking a step into the world of after. I knew because I had been there before.

Almost eleven years earlier, on the morning of November 28, 1993, I woke with a start, a horrible sense of apprehension. As I walked down the hall to my infant son's room, I felt instinctively that it was too quiet. I began to run. Throwing open Jason's door, I knew that I would find him as I did: on his stomach, face down, dead. I remember picking him up, running, screaming, trying to resuscitate him, seeing the fear and disbelief on the faces of my older children. I knew there was no hope.

Within minutes of my husband calling 911, the fire department and police descended on our house, whisking Jason to the nearest emergency room. With bile in my throat, we got in the car and followed, then sat in the waiting room of the hospital, knowing that he was gone. When they finally came to confirm our worst fears, I could hear an agonizing scream come from somewhere deep inside. Our lifeless son was brought to us to say goodbye, his mouth bandaged from the trauma he had sustained during attempts to resuscitate him.

My son Jason, a perfect child in every way, a gift to a family that had already endured tragedy, was dead at five and a half months of age, of sudden infant death syndrome (SIDS). His death was like hitting a wall, no way to get through it, past it or around it. It marked the first invisible boundary in the life of our family, the first before-and-after moment.

Now, in 2004, we were all changed people, a changed family, but we had gone forward, living our lives, having been touched by Jason. With my diagnosis on Friday, August 13, we were about to change again.

On my 40th birthday, three years after Jason died and one year after the much-wanted birth of our son, Matthew, my girlfriends gave me a beautiful luncheon. Many of them had been traumatized at the thought of turning 40. I remember making a speech in which I said that turning 40 was a cakewalk—it was getting to 40 that had been so damn hard.

At 48, facing a diagnosis of cancer, those words echoed inside my head as I wondered if I would make it to 50.

TWO

The first "before and after"

Let me backtrack a little and tell you how I got here. I am Dr. Marla, fashioned to be "Canada's doctor," a role I have enjoyed creating and performing. My passion has been and continues to be medicine—the science, the art, the practice. I cannot remember a time when I did not want to be a doctor. As a little girl, I identified with characters on television who were doctors. I loved people. I loved science . . . it seemed a natural place for me to end up. And it is a decision that I have never regretted. So few people love what they do and who they are. I, in fact, love it all.

Both my parents lived through the Depression years. It made them who they are and determined the kinds of lessons they would teach their two daughters. The first and most important lesson was education, education, education. It was hammered into us from an early age. No one could take away your education. Strive to be the best in whatever you wanted to be. If science was your interest, then reach for the pinnacle of medicine. If language was your interest, strive to become a lawyer. There were no halfway measures in their thinking.

My sister and I are only two years apart, but we are different and diverse people. My sister was formally named Roslyn at birth, but when an older cousin could not pronounce Roslyn, she became Rozzie and then Zozzie. I have known her as Zozzie my entire life. If anyone refers to her as Roslyn, I know that person is remote and does not know her. She is Zozzie. (It is even in the name of the business she has built for herself.)

The diversity of our early years set us apart and kept us apart. My sister is creative and artistic, and though in many ways far smarter than I am, her love was for imagination and design. Mine was always geared toward academic achievement. A university graduate, and now a brilliant designer, she was under-appreciated in those early years because she did not meet what I perceived as the family expectation of getting straight A's. I was the star pupil, and therefore far easier for my parents to relate to. Growing up in the same house with my sister, we might as well have lived in different countries. It must have been hard going to like me in the early years. I was always the standard by which other achievements were measured. It would not be until years later that my sister and I could see each other for who we both are and forge a deep and strong relationship. Now we can joke that I cannot draw a straight line even with a ruler, while Zozzie can create anything with her imagination. Together we are complete.

My mother was a French teacher. In fact she was the one and only specialty French teacher for the upper grades in the public school my sister and I attended. My sister took the option of a teacher who could simply teach the French curriculum, rather than having my mother as a teacher. I, ever the over-achiever who thought that saying no was wrong, rose to the challenge of having my mother, "Madame," teach me French.

She was tough on everyone but tougher on me, aware that the other kids would assume I had an inside track. It was a miserable, almost impossible situation. I couldn't wait to move on to high school.

I started high school at the expected time but, because the courses I wanted weren't available at the lower levels, I found myself accelerating through the curriculum. I completed the requirements for a high-school leaving diploma, which was the Quebec requirement for finishing high school and qualifying for university entrance, graduated top girl in my high school and got an early acceptance to McGill University with a scholarship. I was 15 years old.

I entered McGill University in sciences and by my second year had an early acceptance to McGill's faculty of medicine. I can still remember getting the acceptance into pre-med at McGill. I had just undergone a bilateral surgical procedure to correct kneecaps that refused to stay in place. I had returned home from the Montreal General Hospital in two cumbersome casts, barely able to get around the house. I remember the letter coming, and literally falling over as I read that I had been accepted to medical school. I was 17 years old. It seems like yesterday and, at the same time, a lifetime ago.

I loved medical school, everything about it: the crazy hours, the meticulous memorization. I was on a path to who I wanted to become. I lived, ate and breathed those courses. I let myself be defined by the parameters of who I was being socialized to be: a doctor.

Early on I met the son of friends of my parents who also was in medical school. My parents thought that he could help me navigate the program. David was a few years ahead of me and asked me out. I adored David, but frankly, he was too short for me. As shallow as that seems now, at 18 it seemed to matter. My sister is 5 inches shorter than I am. I introduced her to David, thinking they might be a perfect match. Some 30 years and two fabulous children later, I am still lucky enough to call David my brother-in-law, the father of my niece and nephew and, more important, my friend. When David and Zozzie moved to Baltimore at the end of his residency training, for him to assume a fellowship position at Johns Hopkins, I knew I had lost a substantial part of my family. Yet, while the distance keeps us apart, we have never been closer.

I was surrounded by medicine and doctors, and so it seemed inevitable that I would mostly date doctors. While my social world might have been narrow, I didn't recognize it. In my first year, a girlfriend—not in medical school—fixed me up with Bobby, a recent graduate from textile engineering in Philadelphia. We each knew of the other through mutual friends. He actually stood me up on our first date. (We still argue this point. He, clearly more laid back than I was—or likely could ever be—says we hadn't made firm plans. I, the Rolodex memory kid, knew for a fact we had firm plans.) We did eventually go out on a date and it was instant dislike on my part. I felt he was outside of my world and what was important to me. He was starting his business career and could barely relate to me in medical school with my white knight attitude. It was clear there would be no second date. And there wasn't. Not for another four years, that is.

Medical school consumed me. I had a busy social life with fellow medical students, dated a lot and stayed focused on where I was going. Marriage and family were not in my plans; I never really gave them too much thought. Medicine was what I loved, every aspect of it. What I had grown to love best was the idea of "continuity of care," the term used in the medical field to describe the ongoing, sometimes lifelong, relationship between doctor and patient. And so, despite the prompting of mentors to subspecialize, I forged ahead into family medicine, the most underappreciated role a physician can take.

I graduated with an acceptance into the residency of my choice, family medicine at McGill University. I began to understand that what I was memorizing wasn't about performance on an exam but about performance in real life. Someone, somewhere would one day depend on my diagnostic abilities. I remember being bowled over by the responsibility.

The week after writing my licensing exams, I went to visit friends in Toronto. I was invited to a dinner party, and Bobby was there. Four years older than when we'd last met, he looked entirely different. His business had moved to Toronto, and while he would still have work in Montreal, Toronto was about to become his home. I was just about to start my residency in Montreal. We talked, and exchanged phone numbers.

It seemed like half the medical class was getting married that summer. I went back to Montreal and called Bobby, inviting him to a wedding I had to attend. We had a great time and he didn't seem at all like the man I had met earlier. He had changed. He claims that he hadn't really, that I was one who had changed. Likely it was a bit of both.

We started dating, and to me it seemed perfect. Bobby was commuting between Montreal and Toronto; I was leading the ridiculously busy, sleep-deprived life of an intern. I tried to organize my on-call schedule so that we could see each other on weekends. There were many Sundays when he would pick me up from the hospital and I couldn't stay awake through breakfast.

His entire family had moved to Toronto with the exception of his grandparents, who had stayed in Montreal. On Sunday afternoons when he was in town, he always made time to visit them, even if those hours happened to be the only ones we would have together. His grandparents took precedence. It amazed me how protective and caring he was of them, his incredibly charming grandfather, his somewhat more ornery grandmother. She could not understand why I had to work and would tell me that if I stayed with Bobby he could take care of me. I knew she meant financially, and that it was difficult for her to see that my work was not just work, but also my career and my life. But she was right: Bobby could and did take care of me in the ways that were most important to me. Financially was the least of them.

Bobby was not a physician and a lot of my friends wondered if he could ever "get" me and understand my life. Truth is, I think he is the only one who actually saw me for *who* I was rather than *what* I was. He believed in me, more than I ever believed in myself. He would hang out in the interns' lounge when I was on call and laugh off the guys who would call him Mr. Shapiro. He was and is the most secure person I know. He truly knows who he is. At my most anxious moments, thinking that I could never do it all, he would smile and reassure me that I could be whoever I chose to be. I never quite believed it. I always felt anxious that someone would find me out, that somehow I wasn't good enough, a fraud. I was surrounded by bright, accomplished people. It was intimidating. But I kept plodding ahead, grateful that I could.

Bobby moved to Toronto, I was in Montreal, and we were living out our lives in two different provinces, meeting on weekends. It was hard to remember what clothes I had in each city.

But it allowed me to focus on work and the challenges of being on call and residency training. Ultimately, that was not enough for Bobby. The relationship challenged me to move to Toronto, where he was. Despite trepidation and a marriage proposal that took place on an escalator at Dorval Airport in Montreal, I found myself saying "I do" and moving to Toronto.

Once there, I entered a subspecialty training program in community medicine and epidemiology. I finished my residency program and joined an academic group of physicians at the University of Toronto's Department of Family and Community Medicine. I was a "geographic full-time" (GFT) at the university, splitting my time between seeing patients and training residents. And so I began my life as a practising physician.

It wasn't long until I realized that I could not and would not cope with the frustrations and restraints of being full-time in an academic setting. I loved the teaching, but often the pace was slower than I wanted it to be, and while I truly loved the academics I worked with, I knew it was the wrong time in my life to be there. After my first child was born, I began to wonder if I could open a practice of my own. Bobby would remind me that I was asking the wrong question: the question to ask was not *how* I would do this, but *if* I wanted to. If the answer was yes, then I could find a way. With the support of my husband, who sincerely believed in me, I made the leap into private practice.

In those early days it was so quiet that I sometimes found myself reading magazines between patient visits. But before long the few patients I did have must each have told two friends about me, and they told two friends, and so on . . . I began to be booked months in advance. Who would have known?

And one fateful day a dad showed up with two sick kids. I administered as usual, and before he left I said what I always said, which was to challenge him to confirm that he had really gotten it. Could this dad go home and "be me"? Could he retell my advice with confidence and follow through on it? I have always done this because I believe that unless patients are educated about the why and the what of the advice given, they are not likely to follow through. Incredulously, he asked if I always did that. When I said yes, he smiled and said I should do that on TV. I smiled back and said, "Make me an offer."

Little did I know that an offer was just a breath away. This man, it turned out, was an associate producer for a show called *Cityline* and they were looking for a doctor to replace their departing therapist.

And so a door opened before me that I could not resist. I began my life as a media doctor. I joined CityTV in 1993 as the therapist on *Cityline,* making regular appearances. Instead of being limited to a one-on-one patient relationship, I could "treat" lots of patients all at once. I eventually moved on to health and family day, the news and the all-news station called CP24. I thrived on it, but continued with my first love, the day-to-day practice of medicine. It was busy and only getting busier.

In the meantime, our family life was enduring a series of emotional upheavals and strains. We had two wonderful little girls, but I had also endured a tragic anencephalic pregnancy (in which part of the fetus's brain is congenitally absent) and three subsequent miscarriages. I began to wonder if we would ever have a third child and why I felt the need to keep on trying. But somehow I didn't feel complete. Our family didn't feel complete. Bobby was ready to stop trying, often feeling like a helpless bystander to the havoc being played out in my body. We argued about it but I wouldn't let go, couldn't let go.

Late in 1992, I became pregnant with our first son, Jason. The pregnancy itself was difficult. Because of my history of miscarriages prior to 12 weeks' gestation, I had been labelled a "habitual aborter." The pregnancy this time started smoothly enough, but in my 12th week I started bleeding profusely and a small part of the placenta pulled away from my uterine wall. It happened one weekend up north while my husband and younger daughter were skiing. My elder daughter, who had a case of chicken pox, was stuck at the cottage with me. I remember suffering horrible abdominal discomfort, barely making it upstairs before I realized I was hemorrhaging. I managed to call in Jenna, who at the young age of 8 managed to call some friends, who in turn got me to a local hospital. Jenna wasn't allowed into the ER because she was infectious with chicken pox. She was frightened, I was frightened, but I was stabilized and transferred back to Toronto.

The serial ultrasounds of Jason in utero showed white particulate matter in his bowel, which seemed to indicate the possibility of cystic fibrosis. I thought it was all the blood and protein that he had swallowed from the bleed. Bobby and I underwent genetic counseling and I was flabbergasted to find I was indeed a carrier for CF. Bobby was not. In order for Jason to have inherited CF, both parents would have to be carriers, and then he would have had a one-in-four chance of the disease but a one-in-two chance of being a carrier. We tested him in utero, concerned that the tests might have missed something in Bobby, and he was clear. The pregnancy proceeded uneventfully, but I felt cautious, even anxious.

When Jason was finally born on June 18, 1993, I sighed with the tremendous relief of seeing him healthy, thriving and beautiful. While still on the operating table after the Caesarean section, I had my tubes tied. I had had enough. Jason had been my seventh pregnancy. I thought he would be my last.

As relieved as I was about Jason's safe arrival, I remained uneasy. For reasons I will never understand, I worried about SIDS. It was not a worry I had ever had with the girls, but it was always there with Jason. Call it intuition, a premonition, a sense—whatever prompted it, the concern was always with me.

The night before Jason died, we had given a surprise anniversary celebration for Bobby's parents. My own parents, visiting from Montreal, were staying with us. Jason had a mild cold that night, and earlier that day he had rolled over for the first time. I remember my sense of apprehension that night. The last thing I said to my husband as I went to sleep was, "What if Jason rolls over and dies?" Bobby looked at me as if I were crazy, my anxiety getting the better of me. What-if's are not what is.

In fact, that is exactly what happened. To this day, I recall every moment of my terror as I entered Jason's room the next morning, my powerlessness as I struggled to resuscitate him, the pain of knowing that all my efforts were useless.

When we returned home from the hospital the morning that he died, we discovered that some well-meaning friend had removed all of Jason's pictures. My anger was overwhelming—as if removing his pictures could erase his existence. Shortly thereafter, the police arrived to investigate the death, treating it as a homicide. I remember standing in disbelief, understanding that they were only doing their job, virtually untouched by the invasion of our privacy and the insulting implications. Nothing could possibly be worse than the grief we were all feeling.

Much of what followed—going through the paces of the funeral, the burial and the week of mourning—is like a slow-motion dream. Jason's death was public. I was a public personality and a physician with a full-time practice. I tried to ignore the looks of pity or how the room got quiet when I walked into it. I hated the fact that people were talking about me, about Jason and our family, that I was the topic of the day.

As I went back to work, the office became both a blessing and a curse. Patient after patient felt compelled to say something, never quite knowing what to say. I could sense that some wondered if this could happen to them. It was not that they doubted my competence, but Jason's death had made them realize that even I was not exempt from medical tragedy. It was a frightening message. In fact, I asked myself—hourly—what I could have done differently to keep Jason safe. I could not forgive myself his death, despite all the medical knowledge I had that SIDS is not a preventable event. With my patients, I found myself dissociated from my feelings, performing as a professional, a role that was familiar to me and far easier than the new and excruciating role of the grieving mother. I reassured them that I was fine, and tried to return to the business of their visits. Eventually we put a sign up in the office thanking patients for their concern and good wishes, and providing the address of the fund we had established in Jason's memory.

After the long days were finished, I found myself staring down at my two sleeping daughters, night after night, feeling that only if I watched them breathe could I compel them to stay healthy, to live. Before Jason's death, the girls could go to a friend's house for a sleepover and I wouldn't give their safety a second's thought. Now I had to fight the urge to keep them home with me. I did not want to make them pathologically fearful, and so I would let them go—then spend agonizing hours worrying about them falling down stairs, burning themselves, slipping in a shower, being hit by a car on the street . . . The fears were endless and I could not make them go away.

And it tore me apart to watch my children struggle with the fright and confusion about the loss of their brother. Both girls wondered if they had done something to cause his death. My eldest, Jenna, had celebrated her ninth birthday just a week before his death with a sleepover party, and she wondered—unbeknownst to either Bobby or me at the time—if Jason had caught something at the party that had made him sick and caused his death. Amanda, a mere 6 years old, had been clear about not wanting a baby when we first told her I was pregnant; she wanted to guard her position as the youngest. Though she loved Jason from the minute he was born, she worried that somehow she had wished him away. Both girls were overwhelmed by their feelings of sadness and grief. Neither could understand the horrible sadness they felt and why it was with them from the moment they woke up to when they went to sleep . . . why, in fact, it never left them. Nothing in their young lives could have prepared them for this kind of sadness and confusion. The truth is that nothing in my own life or my professional training could have prepared me for the same kind of feelings I was experiencing.

As a parent, burying my child and coping with my own loss was one element of grief. Coping with my children's grief, realizing I couldn't make it go away, was a life lesson I found so frightening and painful that it took my breath away. It challenged me and Bobby to reach deep inside and find our ability to invite the girls to talk openly about their grief, not deny it. We tried to support them through it and hopefully find ourselves on the other side of it. It was daunting and painful, excruciatingly painful.

The year after Jason's death was, in retrospect, one of the most difficult years of my life. There were times I couldn't breathe. I wondered if it would ever get better. I suffered from terrible insomnia. While I could force myself to function during the day, the nights were interminable. Despite the attempts of my personal physician's prescriptions to get me to sleep, it was clear that I could not let myself sleep and that, until I gave myself permission to sleep again, this was not going to be solved with pills. Nothing but time and mourning were going to get me past this.

At that time I was the on-air doctor for *Cityline,* an hour-long live call-in show. Jason died at the end of November and I was scheduled to do the Christmas show, historically a difficult one that would be filled with calls from people depressed about the season. The producers pulled me off the show, thinking it best to shield me from further sources of depression and grief. I remember being angry and insisting that I do it. Everything in my life felt as if I had lost control, and I wanted to maintain control wherever I could. I would do the show.

I was probably not aware how shocking I looked. I had lost a substantial amount of weight in a short period of time, since eating was not something I had yet remastered. And though the show was difficult, I think it helped me more than it helped any of the callers. It reminded me that life is meant for the living. And I had a decision to make: to return to the land of the living.

I was also beginning to learn the hard lesson that control is an element that we often fool ourselves we have. While we do have the power to make many decisions, so much of life is out of our control. For such a controlled and organized person, that was a bitter pill to swallow.

In the midst of watching my children deal with their incomprehensible grief, I remember feeling that we could not let this defeat us. I had to make my daughters understand that despite terrible grief and tragedy, we were a family without any regrets for Jason's birth, and our love for each other would get us through. I knew, watching my children, that Bobby and I had to go forward and have another child. Not to replace Jason—that was not the message I wanted to give my daughters—but to remind us all about why we had had children in the first place and about all the love we as a family had to share. More than anything, I wanted my children not to be afraid. I wanted them to learn that life—no matter what it gives us—is something to embrace and go forward with, to cope with and, above all, to live.

There was something else too, a more bizarre notion. If something were to happen to me, I reasoned, two siblings were not enough. I have only one sister and we are separated by a great physical distance, living in two different countries. There can be no Friday night dinners, no girl lunches, no schmoozes over coffee. I wanted my daughters to have more than each other if I wasn't there. Perhaps, too, this idea was born out of my daily experience with dying people and unexpected tragedies. I knew that life has no insurance policies, but somehow the idea of having another child seemed like taking out an insurance policy for my children.

Thus it was that I began to investigate the possibility of getting pregnant again. I was on the other side of 35 and had had a tubal ligation at the time of my C-section. Suffice to say this was not going to be easy, and many of my friends and physician colleagues tried to dissuade me. But in this, as in most things in life, I was dogged. My husband knew it was a losing battle to try to talk me out of the physical challenges of getting pregnant.

I felt that although this was, in some ways, selfish, it was also something I had to do—for the girls, myself, my husband. For all of us.

Finding a physician to support me in my attempt to get pregnant was the first difficult task. Many suggested I try in vitro but I knew that was not a route I could take. Having supported many patients through this procedure I knew it would consume me and take me away from the family. While I wanted to have another child, I did not want it to become the sole reason for my moving on in life. I eventually was referred to a physician, an older gynecologist, who empathically listened to my requests. He asked me if I was sure, if we were sure that we were moving ahead for the right reasons. We talked about the surgical challenges I faced, but he was prepared to take the case on. He told me I had to gain some weight and he wanted to see the scale hit the triple digits. We decided not to discuss this with any of our friends or family. I didn't want to be judged or to hear anyone's unsolicited opinion.

The second week in January, a mere seven weeks after Jason died, I found myself in hospital about to undergo an attempt to put me "back together." It felt like the attempt was not only a physical rescue but also an emotional one. And I truly believed that if we did not succeed, I would at least know that we had tried, and that would be a comfort.

The surgery lasted more than five hours. When I awoke I was told that it looked successful, at least on one side. The doctor suggested that I wait two months and then have a hysterosalpingogram, a test where dye is injected into the Fallopian tubes to see if they are open. I declined. I did not want to know. I knew we had done everything possible to restore my fertility. The rest I would leave to fate. In May, I was told to go ahead and try to get pregnant. I had mixed feelings about trying, but on June 18, one year to the day of Jason's birth, I found out I was pregnant.

In February 1995, Matthew was born. It is the custom to name children in my faith after a deceased relative. But Matthew was named after what we felt he was. In Hebrew Matthew means gift from God, and I truly felt we had been given a great gift.

Life continued with us focusing on our children and our families. It was a busy juggling act between family responsibility, car pools, the kids' extracurriculars, the perpetually busy office and my ongoing work on television. We had settled into life with the three kids, and although we missed Jason each and every day, the addition of Matthew to our family brought us endless joy.

In 2000, I was approached by the Canadian Foundation for the Study of Infant Deaths, Health Canada and Procter & Gamble to become the spokesperson for the Back to Sleep Campaign. Tipper Gore had done it briefly in the United States. The campaign was meant to foster a partnership between industry and health. Procter & Gamble, through its Pampers line, had launched a diaper with the words "back to sleep" in two languages to remind parents and other caregivers that infants should be placed only on their backs to sleep. While we did not and do not know what causes sudden infant death syndrome, we know that sleep position can make a huge difference in getting vulnerable SIDS babies through the window of risk.

I went to a joint meeting of the players at the office of a public relations firm to see if I was the right person for the campaign. As I sat there listening to the strategies, it was put to this audience that in fact I might be the wrong person because I already had a "television identity" with the network I was with.

I sat as they debated and suddenly found myself standing up, feeling furious. I looked at this group, realizing that I was nothing other than a face for their campaign, and spoke clearly and loudly. They appeared startled. "Gentlemen, I may be a CityTV personality today, and perhaps I might be another network's personality at some other time, and I might be the face of a campaign for you, but to me, to my family, that is not what we see. Every night when I go to bed, when I wash my face, the person staring me back in the mirror is Jason's mother, a SIDS parent, and no matter what you might see, what the public might see, that is who I see and will always see. I will always be Jason's mother." And with that, I walked out, leaving a somewhat silent room of people who hardly dared move.

I did do the campaign. I wanted to do the campaign and my family was supportive. It would also start a significant friendship in my life. The PR firm connected me with their agent, a man who would be my travelling companion, Scott Morris. Poor Scott had the onerous task of teaching me how to deliver "key messages," a PR term for the most important messages to get out in limited time frames. I would stare him down, telling him I had lived the key messages and that there was not much he was going to teach me about messaging and on-air appearances. I knew that Pampers wanted to sell diapers, but they had a great message and a great cause, and I was grateful to P & G for an important campaign. I wanted to sell the message. I had no qualms bringing my diapers with me across the country.

And across the country we did go. Radio stations, television, newspapers . . . I was tireless and wanted to keep each interview as fresh as the previous one. I wanted the message out there. I talked endlessly about my own tragedy and listened endlessly to other tragic SIDS stories. In many small communities across the country there are no support groups, and I listened to the same fears and questions over and over again from parents who wondered what they had done wrong to lose an apparently normal child.

By the time we hit the east coast, I was beginning to lose it. The emotional baggage I was lugging with me was getting heavier and more difficult to carry. We returned to Toronto, to an appearance on *Canada AM* at CTV. I told Jason's story on air to Dan Matheson and reviewed what parents could do to reduce their risk of SIDS.

I immediately felt comfortable on the set of *Canada AM*. By that time, Scott was encouraging me to change networks to a larger venue. The only place I wanted to go was CTV. Jason's death opened that door. While I could have opened it myself, it felt as though he were beside me.

Canada AM was in the midst of changing executive producers. The current executive producer, Michael Serapio, introduced me to the incoming executive producer, Jordan Schwartz. Over coffee, the three of us exchanged ideas about the development of a consistent on-air medical position, a person whom viewers could turn to and trust to explain the medical news and what it meant to them. Jordan wanted to create a group of on-air specialists. Unlike the work I had been doing at *Cityline,* it would be more focused on breaking medical news. I loved his vision. I was excited about the opportunity to expand into medical news and create the role of a medical contributor. I joined the *Canada AM* family in September 2000.

During my seven years at *Cityline* I had established a wonderful relationship with the producers and directors. They were proud and excited for me. They wished me every opportunity for success and growth. The host, Marilyn Denis, had become a close friend. She is an elegant woman, a funny person and a supportive friend; that friendship has endured. Who I was on television or who I might become had nothing to do with who we were as people. Marilyn, as always, was wonderful, understanding what this new opportunity at CTV would offer me. As my friend, she encouraged me and celebrated with me. As my boss on *Cityline,* she told me she would miss my contribution. As nervous as I was, she more than anyone threw me out the door, telling me to "go get 'em."

Within a year at *Canada AM* I was asked to start doing the weekend medical updates on our all-news station, Newsnet. And, on occasion, when the story merited, I was asked to do a talkback on the national news at 11 p.m.

Every time a health or lifestyle story appeared on the set, whether on nutrition or exercise, I would nudge Jordan in the side and tell him how I would ask it differently, better, what was missing. We joke that he got tired of me bruising his ribs. In 2002 he asked me if I wanted to host a new talk show, a daily 30-minute health and lifestyle program. It would be called *Balance . . . television for living well.*

Hosting a talk show is different from being the medical expert. All of a sudden you are in the driver's seat, forging ahead with the interview, responsible for getting it on time to commercial, making sure the interview is entertaining and interesting. This was not as easy as it looked, believe me! And of course, I gave up nothing else: *Canada AM,* Newsnet, the national news, my full-time practice. It was busy. Every night the three kids and I would sit down and do homework, me reading books, scripts. It was a ton of work. And my husband, who clearly was not so thrilled to lose his wife completely to her career, knew that this was something I had to do. For the first time ever, he was driving carpool. Mr. Mom. I could not have done any of this without Bobby's help.

Balance was an amazing experience. I met fascinating people, read dozens, maybe hundreds, of books, and expanded my areas of interest. It made me a better doctor, more open to alternative care. Dr. Andrew Weil taught me about integrative medicine; Dr. Phil, well, showmanship at its best; Delta Burke, depression under a microscope. And so Dr. Marla was born.

During season two, I went to New York to interview Dr. Sanjay Gupta on the set of *American Morning* at CNN. I envied his team of producers in medical news, his ongoing coverage of breaking stories. And although he graciously pointed out the similarities in what we both did, the differences were glaringly obvious to me.

I also had the opportunity to interview talk-show host Meredith Viera and her husband, Richard Cohen. Richard suffers from multiple sclerosis and had fought two bouts of colon cancer. (His book, *Blindsided,* a how-to book on coping with chronic illness, would become an inspiration as my own battle with cancer began.)

The second season of *Balance* had been frustrating and difficult. The Canadian elections required that we give up our set earlier than anticipated, as it was needed for election coverage. I found myself doing 10 shows a week, running my practice and still trying to maintain a semblance of family life. When the season was over, I didn't miss it as I had season one. I was also frustrated with my role on *Canada AM,* wanting to do more medical news and reporting. So when ABC presented an offer to be on *Good Morning America* I was not only flattered, I wanted the job. I was ripe for another change. But it would mean being on an airplane every week. And it would also mean leaving *Balance*. There I was, weighing the pros and cons, in the middle of a negotiation that I knew could change my life immeasurably.

Life was exciting. The kids were doing well, Bobby was busy at work developing new projects, and he would be going to China in late summer with the Canadian business delegation. I was enjoying being on hiatus. Then again, hiatus for me meant the office, *Canada AM* and Newsnet.

The proverbial other shoe was about to drop.

THREE

Superstition and reality

August 13, a Friday. Seems scripted, doesn't it? But it isn't. That's the day I joined a club that up until now I had been a supporter of . . . the breast cancer club. A club I had no desire to be a member of. I had a mammogram and ultrasound booked. My last one had been 18 months earlier, so it was a good time for me to go. I had always had very dense breasts (which essentially means there is not much fat), and I knew that made it harder to get a clear picture of the glandular tissue in a mammogram. So, despite always having normal mammograms and no family history of breast cancer, I had still been concerned about breast cancer. It is impossible to do what I do for a living and not let such concerns creep in on a personal level.

Several years earlier I had started going to a respected breast surgeon, Dr. David McCready, for my exams. Though I had had intermittent cysts, there had never been anything serious, and he always wondered why I came to him. What he was really saying, I knew, was that his time was valuable and I didn't need him. But as a fellow physician he tolerated my visits and was able to reassure me that all was well. Somewhere inside, I must have known I would need him.

As I came out after my films were done, the standard views that are undertaken in a routine mammogram, the radiologist (not my usual radiologist, but someone I didn't know well) asked me to stay for a magnification view. She wanted to take a second look at an area of "indeterminant calcifications." Calcifications are not unusual, and they are often benign and of no importance. On occasion, however, they are classic in their appearance and the signs of underlying malignant disease.

I went back in. I waited. The radiologist came out to the area where I had been asked to wait at the back of the hallway, and couldn't look me in the eye. She told me she couldn't be sure of anything, but thought I should have a core biopsy. I knew I was in trouble, more by her manner than anything else.

Core biopsies are a relatively new procedure. They are designed to help eliminate unnecessary surgical procedures. When an ultrasound identifies a solid mass that is suspicious or a mammogram image identifies an area of calcification that is indeterminate, a core biopsy is done as an intermediary procedure. My breast abnormality was seen on mammography rather than by ultrasound. A stereotactic core would find the calcifications seen on the film, and biopsy them. To do this, the patient stands upright and each breast is held in place, flattened like a pancake, much as is done in a routine mammogram. The film is used as a map, a guide to where and how deep the calcifications are. Then, in a five-pointed star pattern, tissue is removed and examined to reach a diagnosis.

On that Friday the 13th, the radiologist was recommending I get this done. Quickly.

I got dressed, walked next door to Princess Margaret Hospital, and asked to interrupt my surgeon. He assumed I was there to ask about mutual patients. I quickly told him I was in trouble, and passed on what the radiologist had said. He was going on vacation that afternoon, but I told him I would organize everything and see him, hopefully with the results of the core biopsy, when he returned on August 30.

I went home, worried and anxious. My gut told me I was in trouble. I *was* in trouble.

I had to hold my breath until Wednesday, when the core biopsy was booked, wondering what bad news it would have for me. None of this could happen quickly enough for me.

Getting through the weekend was murder. I didn't know where to throw myself. We went to a movie Saturday night with two friends—friends who know me well and would see that I was out of sorts. I told them both. I widened the circle of confidentiality by telling my sister-in-law Wendy, who has always been a close friend and confidante. I confided in my girlfriend Susan, who insisted she would go with me to the biopsy, that this would all be no big deal, that I was a doctor and they were being extra cautious. And although I had told myself the same things, I knew they weren't true. The sixth sense that has always been with me, both as a physician and in my own life, was not sending me good messages.

We arrived at Princess Margaret on Wednesday, August 18, for the core biopsy. The chief of radiology, Dr. Marcus Dill-Macky, entered the examination room and asked if I had seen my films. Together, we reviewed them. He talked about the films as if they didn't belong to me. Cheerily, assuredly, he showed me the area in question, telling me it was a classic finding of malignancy, likely a ductal carcinoma. It measured 1.6

centimetres and, in the best-case scenario, would turn out to be a low-grade malignancy, in situ. The best kind of cancer to have, if you will. It actually was fascinating—the problem was that these were *my* breasts, not someone else's. As we got up to prepare me for the core biopsy, I popped my head into the waiting room and told Susan that if there had been any doubt, it had been erased. I had cancer. She looked a little stunned; I felt stunned, but as if this really were not me at all. *Surely it must be someone else's breasts he was talking about.*

I went into the room where the biopsy would take place. As I expected, the nurse told me I had to do this in an upright position. And, similar to a mammogram, my breast was locked into a pancake position to hold it in place. Using the x-ray machine they would create a three-dimensional image of my breast and the calcifications, which were the most likely markers of disease. These calcifications could be seen only in the images on the films and were not palpable—that is, they couldn't be felt. The computer-generated images would create a road map of how far the punch biopsy should go to capture the calcifications. The doctor froze the area, made a small incision at his point of entry and then, with five loud, gun-like bangs, he cored out the areas of suspicion. He told me I would need MRIs of my breasts before the surgery. He asked me if I wanted to enter a study looking at the difference between doing MRIs of both breasts simultaneously versus one breast at a time. I silently nodded my consent, and got dressed.

Susan and I walked out and got into her car. I am not sure what exactly I was thinking. My husband called my cell; there had been six calls from him. I knew he was sitting on pins and needles. I heard his voice and started to cry. I gave Susan the phone. She repeated what I told her the radiologist had told me. I asked her to call my sister in Baltimore and tell her. I stopped crying. I looked at Susan in disbelief. How could this be happening? It really didn't matter how. It was.

I went home and waited for Bobby. He was devastated but calm, and reminded me we had gotten through a lot before and we would get through this too. I was angry. I knew there was a "we" here—that this would affect all of us—but really this was me. And all I could think of was that I was going to die. Despite the hundreds of women I had taken care of with breast cancer over the years, many of whom had fared well, all I could think about were the women who had died.

I realized that my reaction was like every other woman's, except that I could not reassure myself—even though, in my job, I reassure men and women all day long. There is no reassurance for a physician. We know too much. We see it all. I knew my breasts were dense. I knew the cancer had been there a year ago, but because of the density could not be seen. Knowledge, in this case, was devastating and chilling.

We waited a couple of days. Bobby was going to China the following week. We decided that even though we didn't have the final pathology we would tell the girls. Girls? They were young women. Jenna was eight weeks away from her 20th birthday, Amanda was 17½ and entering her last year of high school. We decided not to tell Matt—he was only 9. We sat down with Jenna and Amanda and sounded optimistic as we told them this was small and had been caught early. I tried to believe the words coming out of my mouth. My sister-in-law Wendy was with us. We told them that we wanted to keep this quiet, that I wasn't willing to talk about this publicly, at least not now, but that they could ask us whatever they needed to, whenever they needed. I would hide nothing from them. I would be fine. I had to be fine. Tears came to their eyes, but I sounded supremely confident and it seemed to help. I didn't feel all that confident but I needed to be, for them.

We made it through the weekend. Life seemed normal, but every once in a while I rode a wave of terror that seemed to come over me without notice. I tried to mask it, reminding myself I did not know enough. But I knew too much.

Monday morning, I received a phone call from Dr. Karina Bukhanov, the colleague and radiologist who had done my previous mammograms, but who had been away when the latest films were done. We had shared many cases over the years and I had grown to trust and respect her judgment. I had left a message for her that Friday when the first mammogram was done. Now, just back from vacation, she had no idea what was happening. I filled her in, and she said she would call me right back. Fifteen minutes later she called, the concern in her voice obvious. She told me it was an aggressive ductal carcinoma, a grade 3 out of 3, the most aggressive of cell types. Worst of all, the pathologist who had read the slides thought there might be micro-invasion, which meant a more advanced stage of cancer. Unlike the hopeful thought that this would be confined to the duct alone, it appeared that the tumour had invaded the duct. I could feel myself stop breathing as she spoke.

With this information, the next step, I knew, would be an MRI (magnetic resonance imaging). MRIs are difficult to arrange in Canada, with lengthy waiting times, unlike in the United States. Patients often ask me why they can't have an MRI as part of an investigation; everyone sees new technology as the panacea. The fact is that MRI often is not as good as routine mammography for finding cancers. While MRI has been proven to be a very valuable tool in certain populations (such as women who are carriers of the genes BRCA1 and BRCA2), it is not for everyone. To date, while MRI is sensitive in finding about 90% of invasive cancers, it is only 50% successful in detecting ductal carcinoma in situ. In addition, breast MRI is difficult to perform well. A unit has to have a dedicated breast coil with special sequences to darken whatever fatty tissue there is, or to subtract one set of images from the other. Last, and important in our medical system, breast MRI is expensive relative to mammography or breast ultrasound. Even in the United States, where there are so many scanners, there is the issue of insurance carriers and whether they will pay for it. Certainly this is not a test to replace routine mammography, but an additional tool that should be used for selected at-risk patients. With breasts as dense as mine, and even without a family history of breast cancer, I should have been offered an MRI as an additional routine screening tool. I could feel the anger welling up in me at this thought.

But now, having a confirmed diagnosis of breast cancer, I needed the MRIs. It was possible the MRIs would give us more information that the mammograms had missed. We knew that the mammogram had missed my cancer when it was there one year earlier. Were there more problem areas lurking?

The MRIs were arranged for September 8, 13 and 15, with the surgery on September 16 (my surgeon was away when I called to arrange the surgery date, but I knew enough not to wait for his return to book with his secretary; I had played this game of shortening wait times all too often on behalf of my patients). Still, I worried that if the MRI on September 15 showed something else, there would not be time to investigate it and the surgery would be delayed. I felt that a month was an eternity to wait, although I knew that in the Canadian health care system it was actually timely. Karina told me she would get the right breast MRI moved up, if possible, to get a clearer picture, and she found a time for me two days later, on Wednesday, August 25.

I tried to focus. I had a full office. I told my secretary Barb as I walked out. She knew I had been on the phone with Dr. Bukhanov. I repeated the news that it was a ductal carcinoma and it looked invasive; it was not confined to just the duct. She looked incredulous and asked how that could be. I cut her off. I said, "Don't—that doesn't help." And she of all people. She had just finished her own issues with breast cancer. If anyone knew, it was her. Despite her own battles with the disease, it was shocking and upsetting for Barb that this could happen to me, her doctor, her friend, a woman she saw keeping everyone healthy. I was not supposed to get this disease. But is anyone?

I went through the day, "third-spacing" this information, pushing it to the back of my mind, pretending it wasn't me. But it was me. *It is me,* I thought. *I have breast cancer and it isn't looking good.*

This was Monday. The MRI was booked for Wednesday. Bobby was to leave for China on Thursday and I with the kids for a getaway to Chicago, since the kids had not been together all summer. I wanted to carry on, I wanted us to go through with our plans. Bobby was torn but I told him there was no reason for him not to go, that I wanted him to go. We all packed for our departures on Thursday, none of us quite understanding how we felt. First, though, there was the MRI.

I had entered a study on simultaneous dynamic bilateral breast imaging in MRI. It's a mouthful but less complicated than it sounds. The study was designed to use a new breast-imaging protocol and compare it to the existing protocol. Because of technical constraints, the norm had been to do one MRI scan at a time, one breast at a time. A new technology allowed both breasts to be scanned simultaneously. If accurate, the benefits were obvious. But the accuracy of the test had to be compared to the standard tests. It seemed reasonable to participate and I knew that patients under study are often moved through the system faster.

I went for the MRI on Wednesday, alone because I had not allowed anyone to accompany me. I had slipped into that role between patient and doctor. The people checking me in told me how much they loved the show. None of this felt real. I rolled over, undressed on the narrow MRI table. This test is not for the claustrophobic. I lay, face down, with my hands placed over my head in a diver's position. On a plate with two holes cut out, I placed my breasts through the holes, with a nurse pulling and positioning them. I felt like a cow with my udders dangling. The nurse blew the first two punctures for the intra-venous, nervous because she was working on me, a well-known doctor. Dr. Dill-Macky, the radiologist doing the study, entered the room and assured me he was the best. I smiled at him that I *needed* the best. He started the IV and closed the line with saline. They would use this as a portal to inject gadolinium. The MRI is first done without any dye (called the dynamic phase) and then, while the dye is injected, the MRI examines the breasts (the progressive phase).

The table I was lying on was slid inside the MRI machine, the tube so narrow that my arms touched the sides. It felt claustrophobic, like being in a coffin. I had plugs in my ears because the noise of the MRI is deafening. I had been given a buzzer to ring in an emergency. I tried to control my breathing; I tried not to move. I wanted to be a good patient.

The whole procedure took an hour or so—an eternity. I was released, but everyone had gone. There was no one to talk to. It was now after hours and the hallways were completely empty. It was hot; I felt dizzy and anxious. I got dressed and left the hospital to hail a cab; there was none.

I have refused to let my friends come with me for this, another sign of how much I want this not to be happening. This is not a role I want to play. I am the person who makes people better. I am the person everyone comes to. I am the person who gives support, offers hope. I give, I don't take. I don't want to take. I am clear that I want to do this alone. I have to do this alone.

The few friends I had told weren't sure what to do with me. Two of them sounded normal, which I appreciated. The other two had that tone, that horrible empathic tone that made me want to reach through the phone and kill them. I knew they were trying to help, wanted to help. But I explained to them in no uncertain terms that this was not helping. Calling me three times a day with that tone just reinforced my sense that they pitied me and were certain I was going to die. Their offers to bring me dinner infuriated me: I had cancer; I had not lost my ability to cook. And I felt fine, I felt well. Nothing had changed—except everything had changed. I was angry. And although my anger was directed at them I knew enough to know that I was just angry. Period. Anger is easier to deal with than fear and grief. Hey, I'd read *On Death and Dying.* I knew all that. But somehow knowing didn't make me any less angry. I was furious.

My girlfriends insisted on coming over. They brought dinner, we drank wine, we laughed. I didn't feel like me. I didn't feel any different but I knew that everything was different. I felt like I had started the process of dying.

The next morning the whole family piled into a stretch limo. Bobby dropped us off first at our terminal, on our way to Chicago. He was on his way to China via Vancouver. He was torn, but I told him to go. He needed to go. We needed to live our lives.

I arrived in Chicago with the kids and turned my cellphone on. There was a message from Dr. Dill-Macky. In his matter-of-fact way he asked me to call him. I could barely dial the numbers. He told me the tumour was not 1.6 centimetres, as first thought. The MRI showed enhancement of 4.6 centimetres. He told me it was all along the duct, this 4.6-centimetre area, so it was likely all tumour. I was dumbfounded, breathless. I also appreciated his candour and frankness: I needed to know, even though I didn't like what I was hearing. That was not all. There was something in the left breast. The mammogram didn't show what the MRI was showing in the left breast, nor did the ultrasound. It was likely nothing but it needed further investigation. I wondered how I would ever make it through the weekend in Chicago. I was there with a girlfriend from the network. We looked at each other, not really believing any of this but determined that we would all have a good time.

I managed to stay in the moment most of the time, enjoying my children. But I couldn't help letting my mind go to that dark place. Matt was nine years old. *He is only nine. How can I lose him, he lose me?* I was terrified, utterly and totally terrified.

In Chicago I connected with Art Smith. Art is Oprah's chef, a wonderful man who has been on *Balance* several times. I adore him. He is a giving man with a huge heart. He has started an organization called Common Threads, which teaches under-privileged children about life, culture, nutrition and so much more through food and cooking. He offered to pick us up and have dinner. It was a welcome distraction. We met him downstairs and when I got into his car he gave me a chef's outfit for a project he had just been involved in on breast cancer. I could barely breathe. I dared not turn around and look at my girlfriend. This was hitting too close to home.

I managed to make it through the weekend. I was finally going to see my surgeon, David McCready, the next day, Monday, August 30. Bobby was still in China, of course, and so I made the hard decision to take my daughters with me for the appointment. They had made it clear that they wanted to be part of this and that they were adults in their own right. They picked me up at the office and we headed downtown to the Princess Margaret Hospital. I had mixed feelings. So many people look ill there, and I didn't want to scare the girls. But this was my reality. This was their reality.

In the waiting room, I was recognized by some other women; I could hear them wondering why I was there. Though I was polite, I offered up nothing. Finally, David's nurse called me in. And finally he walked in. I was so grateful to see him at last. This was the only person I wanted to talk to. I needed to hear what he thought. I wanted a plan. I *needed* a plan. And suddenly I realized what I mean to my patients. It is an awesome responsibility, and one I have never taken lightly, but never before had it been so clear to me.

He was quiet as he looked at the data. He is not one to be rushed. And despite my telling him to take off both breasts—a demand he hears all the time—he reminded me that we did not have all the data. The right breast, where we had "known burden of disease," was to be his focus during the surgery, but until he had all the pathology and was clear about the question of invasion, he would not do a mastectomy. I worried that he would not get it all, that mine was not a palpable tumour, that it was only visible (and incompletely, at that) on the mammogram.

We discussed the issue of going after lymph nodes. He was ambivalent, given that it was not yet known if there was invasion, and taking out the nodes would pose an unnecessary risk. I could be left with lymphedema, a condition in which there is permanent swelling of the arm because the drainage system—the lymph nodes—has been removed. Prior to the operation, they would localize the centre of the calcification, putting in a hook much as though hooking a fish. I had used this term a hundred times with my own patients and suddenly I realized that I didn't really know how it was done. The experts, I've always said, will be far better at explaining than I can be. Now, with myself as the patient, I wondered what this was really about. David said that I would be taken to the OR and the duct would be dissected following the parameters suggested by the MRI. After much deliberation he decided that, given the size of the tumour on the MRI, the aggressive grade of 3 and the suggestion of invasion, he would go after a few sentinel nodes.

This is a relatively new procedure: instead of taking all the nodes in the armpit, he would have me injected with methylene blue dye or radioactive particles directly into the breast tissue where the tumour was thought to be, and the lymph nodes that drained the area would pick up these injectable particles. Hopefully only a few nodes would show up in imaging studies; he would take those out. The sentinel nodes are thought to be the primary and most important nodes that drain the breast; if there was spread, there was a 95% chance that we would find the spread there. There was also that 5% chance that it might have spread to the lymph nodes but would be missed by this technique, but this is what my surgeon felt was most reasonable. I had to get out of the driver's seat and let him drive. This was hard for me, but I forced myself to relinquish decision-making to him. We agreed that we would wait for the final pathology report before we decided if more surgery was needed, or chemo, or radiation. He was trying to keep me focused. I was trying to stay focused.

We discussed the left breast and he shrugged: he could not remove what he could not see or feel, and perhaps it would be best to follow up with frequent MRIs. Radiology had suggested we do a few more views and a targeted ultrasound to see if we could sort it out. My nature is such that I need a definitive answer, and I was determined that we find a way to get that tissue out as well. David reminded me to concentrate on the right breast, where there was known burden of disease. We use that phrase often in medicine. He was right: this disease was indeed a burden and I wanted it out.

I asked him about travelling. I had so many speaking engagements booked—and ABC: what should I do with the ABC negotiations? He asked me what my priorities were. I looked at him and told him that two of my priorities were sitting in his waiting room; the other priority was only nine and he was at home. He told me to put the contract negotiations on hold. I asked him to say hello to the girls, even though I knew that I had taken a ton of his time and he was running late. He looked at me and said, "You have been coming here for years." I smiled and said that somehow I had always known I would need him, but that even with vigilance and magical thinking, I was in deep trouble with a tumour that was more advanced than I wanted to admit. He nodded and came out to the waiting room to meet the girls, understanding that they needed to put a face to their mother's doctor, and we got ready to leave. I signed the consent for surgery.

Jenna and Amanda and I headed over to Mount Sinai for a meeting with my radiologist, Dr. Bukhanov. We were all doing our best to hold everything together. I was doing my best to stay calm so that the girls would be calm and feel that there was a plan in place, a team who would make me well. I knew that Karina was by my side—she really did get this. She deals with women all day long, since mammography and its related tests are her area of expertise. She did another ultrasound of the left breast, finding the area that she thought would marry up to the suspicious area seen on the MRI. She saw nothing other than a cyst and attempted to aspirate it. She thought it looked all right, but planned to do another MRI in two days and see what a single MRI of the breast looked like. She understood that I could not be easily reassured, that I needed a more definitive answer. I pointed out the obvious: she and I knew that by the time we diagnose breast cancer—even so-called early breast cancer—it has already been there for some time, avoiding detection.

The girls and I headed home. I reminded them that it would be okay. It would be fine.

I coasted through the next 48 hours. Bobby was still in China and we were communicating over the Internet and through brief phone calls. I tried to sound upbeat. There was no point in making him any crazier than I knew he already felt.

Wednesday, September 1, and time for MRI number two.

An e-mail from my brother-in-law early in the day alerted me to the fact that my sister, Zozzie, had told her daughter about my diagnosis. At 23, my niece is an adult, but I was outraged that my sister had told her without asking me. I was supposed to visit Zozzie in Baltimore over the Labour Day weekend but now I couldn't decide if I wanted to go. My anger was out of proportion to the event and I realized that I was emotionally on a very short wire, very thin ice. I was clearly cracking.

Jenna drove me to the hospital for my next MRI. I was hit by a wall of anxiety. Unexpectedly, I found myself doing what I most wanted to avoid: I started to cry in Jenna's car, weeping and pouring out my fear that I would die. I realized how wrong this was, how much I was panicking her, but I could not stop. She was calmer than I; she seemed to understand the fear and reassured me I would be okay. I wanted to believe her. I know there is no place for negative thinking.

Karina Bukhanov and I had agreed that we would do a single MRI of the left breast, the "healthy" breast with that area of uncertainty. Again I lay face down, was injected with gadolinium and, 45 minutes later, was released. This was beginning to feel familiar.

I headed home, fragile and anxious. I had tickets to go to *Canadian Idol* with my kids. The producers were expecting me, and had arranged a backstage tour for the kids. They planned to show me on air with my name and the name of the show, *Balance*—great PR for the launch of our new fall season. I stepped into the shower, hoping to wash off the experience of the MRI. The phone rang—it was Bobby from China. I heard his voice and fell apart. Hopelessly sobbing, I was barely coherent. I felt awful. He was so far away, and I was sobbing how alone I felt, how hard it was at night. I did indeed need him to be home. Falling apart like this seemed so foreign to me, and I realized how much of the time I define myself as a professional—I began wondering if I knew myself at all.

I hung up, put on my Dr. Marla face and headed downtown. The show was a great distraction, and as my face was flashed across the nation I wondered if I looked any different from who I was less than a month ago. I sure felt different.

I still didn't know if I would go to Baltimore; I couldn't make up my mind. I realized my anger at my sister was misplaced. We call it transference in medical lingo. In other words, it was easier to be mad at her than to face my fear. Anger is a familiar emotion, while fear, on the other hand, is foreign and terrifying. I laughed at myself, able to explain it all but unable to control it or make it go away.

I called my sister and spoke to her husband, who is also a physician. His earlier e-mail had asked if my sister had gotten the information wrong when she told him that the tumour was nearly 5 centimetres. Surely she meant 5 millimetres? No, I told him over the phone, she was right: it was indeed close to 5 centimetres, and his e-mail sure hadn't helped. He was mortified at what he had written. I tried to tell him what this felt like. He understood, having lost his mother to ovarian cancer and a stepsister in her forties to breast cancer. I decided to get on the plane to Baltimore. Late that night, I was packing for myself and Matt, hoping that the weekend away would make the time pass.

FOUR

You can fly but you can't hide

I cleared off my e-mail and laughed at another girlfriend's electronic missive. I was glad to be laughing. Renee . . . she is a wonderful friend. She and I usually catch each other early in the morning online and chat briefly over the Internet. I tend not to talk a lot on the phone, given all my work commitments, but since my diagnosis the phone calls from friends had been making me nuts. I had warned them all to back off and stop calling me. Renee wrote in reply:

Mar,

I really do understand your wishes . . . This is all so strange. I know that besides our morning "messaging" at 6 AM it is weird to speak so frequently. And I really do struggle with whether or not to bother you. But as much as I think of you often (and always have) as I flip the channel on my TV everyday, I think of you more now. And the reality is, that is the way life is . . . at least as the caring people that we both are. Old friends who love each other and have always been there for each other and always will be. I certainly can't provide you with any medical support or informed advice, as you have always done for all of us. There are others certainly for that. But I will always be there to provide any support that I can, and I know that you know that. And you will never ask for my help, because it is in me to be there anyways. Besides, I never feel that I am helping, but only sharing, as we have before through all our joys and frustrations and sorrows and many, many secrets! Actually, it makes me feel better to share this with you, and so, in many ways, it is a very selfish act. I am certain that the frequent calls and the questions just make it more difficult and are nothing short of bothersome and annoying. I also imagine that at times you want nothing to do with anyone, while at others you do want to talk and vent. Sometimes it can be someone you're close to, at other times someone more distant. I will always be here to listen when you want. But the truth is the choice as to how you handle this and with whom is yours entirely. I would never want to appear intrusive. You know that. The reality is it is a real struggle to decide whether to call, or just to somehow wait to "hear" how you are doing. I think you can understand that.

I ask myself what I would want in this situation, and I have to be honest and say that I could not even imagine being in your shoes. I would be an idiot to think I could. I do know though that I also like to function independently and would probably also want to do things on my own. I also know that when I am with you and my other friends who mean so much to me, although I may initially resist the attention, the worst things do seem a little better. I guess that is what I hope I can do for you. I wish you a wonderful trip. I will respect your "back off" wishes and understand all you are saying. But please remember that I have a case of Yellow Tail waiting, whenever and for any reason at all. And you know I love you.

Kisses,
Renee

Reading this e-mail at the end of the weekend in Baltimore, I reminded myself how lucky I was to have all these friends. But I also found myself wondering if they would all be there for my kids if I was not. I had to force myself to stop going down that self-indulgent road. I turned off the lights and tried to sleep. Sleep—that precious commodity—constantly eluded me.

The weekend in Baltimore had proven to be helpful in that Matt and I could "hang" together without the distraction of his friends and a basketball net! My sister was warm, but we didn't talk about the breast cancer. I love to shop but was not interested in shopping, and she was concerned. I tried hard. My niece joked that I dress for style and my sister dresses for comfort. It felt odd to have Zozzie push me towards the malls.

Over the weekend I had picked up another voicemail from my radiologist saying that the MRI showed the left breast lesion to be "progressive." I couldn't imagine how that was good but in the message she told me that she thought it indicated only fibrous changes. She also told me that there is a way to localize it with MRI. But it was Labour Day weekend and I could not talk to her. Again I found myself holding my breath. And I could not help but imagine all those cancer cells multiplying, invading. I could not get over the fact that surgery was still another two weeks away. More than anything I wanted it to be over. And I felt calm about the idea of removing both breasts. I could imagine my surgeon, David, telling me how irrational that was at this stage, but I knew that the tumour in the right breast had been there a year ago but not picked up on mammogram. I could not help worrying about what else might be lurking there, unseen.

I became anxious every time I looked at my kids. More than anything I wanted to live, to be there for them and with them. The weekend passed and I managed to get through. On the way to the airport I felt the anxiety beginning to wash over me. I looked at my sister to say goodbye and the tears started to flow. Wordlessly, I turned away and headed towards the check-in.

E-mails kept coming about my speaking engagements and I answered them methodically and professionally. I couldn't help but feel that there were two of me, and I wondered when the me with breast cancer would catch up with the healthy me and I would have to cancel promised appearances. The network had asked me to go to Vancouver to appear on Vicki Gabereau's talk show to promote the new season of *Balance*. I made excuses. I was not ready to tell them the truth yet. I felt that I was being less than honest but I was not prepared to share this yet; I was not ready to become the poster child for breast cancer. Not yet. Not when the whole picture was still eluding me. I didn't know what I was facing in terms of treatment and, at any rate, this was to be a private passage.

I knew that somewhere along the line I *would* want to talk about this, to share my experiences—perhaps doing so would help someone. I was not sure who that might be—me or an anonymous someone out there experiencing the same thing. I had not told my parents yet and I could not imagine how I would. They hate speaking on the phone because they have difficulty hearing, and I could not send this news in an e-mail. Until I knew what I was facing I couldn't fathom telling them. Bobby's mother lives in Toronto and we are close. She is the grandparent the kids know so well, given that Bobby's dad, a man we all loved so dearly, died of melanoma a few years earlier. I dreaded telling her I had cancer. These were all parents and grandparents who had buried a grandson, an event that is not in the normal progression that life should follow. They all would have the same questions I had, questions that I did not have answers to. No, I could not talk about this yet, not until I knew the whole story.

While we were waiting to know more, I spent the time trying on scenarios for size. I would have to make the decision about radiation versus a mastectomy. I knew my surgeon was in favour of breast-conserving surgery. Over the years I had seen countless women who had had mastectomies. And yes, the appearance is shocking, but as a physician I was not married to my breast. It occurred to me, *I am a woman as well, but clearly I have identified myself as a physician for so long that it overshadows any other thoughts, pushing them to the back of my mind. It is easier for me to think as a clinician than as a woman. If I honestly believe that a mastectomy will increase my chances of survival, that is what I will choose.* I tried on the thought of a double mastectomy. There was always the option of reconstruction. I had nursed many patients through the discomfort of tissue expanders placed under the skin to

48

stretch it out to make space for an implant to be placed and gradually inflated with saline. I tried not to go there.

My mind shifted to the issue of micro-invasion. My gut was telling me that the tumour would show invasion, or at least micro-invasion, at the centre. I knew that if there were no invasion at the margins I would be dissuaded from chemotherapy. But I knew that I would err on the side of caution and go with chemotherapy if it was an option. I was 48 years old. I was not interested in waiting to see if this would recur. I did not want a local recurrence and I didn't want spread—metastases—to my bones, brain or liver. My gut was telling me that the first go-round is the best, most effective go-round, but that was not based on science. As a physician I knew there was not necessarily enough evidence to support my point of view. I was also aware that the choice for chemo would be given only if it was a reasonable option: I could not sell the idea if it was not truly merited. But if offered, I would take it. And I realized that if I went that route, my treatment would become obvious, visible, and I would have to go public. I would have outed myself, so to speak.

I told myself that I was being unreasonable. I was the patient, not the doctor. I had to sit back and listen. I do understand the value of evidence, and know that it's the only way we have made any progress in medicine. Flying by your gut is not the way to go in medicine and I realized that the fear in my gut had been doing all the talking.

I tried to talk to myself as I talked to my patients. There was nothing to be gained from what-if scenarios. It is always better to deal with what is. But I didn't know what was and the uncertainty was making me anxious, more anxious than I'd ever thought possible. I couldn't imagine being more anxious.

Yet at work and on air, I was able to perform. It was so much easier to assume that professional role. I felt safe and protected in that role.

I was doing my best not to be angry. But I was angry. *How can I have a tumour that is so large? How can I know as much as I do, be as vigilant as I am and still find myself where I am?* My anger boiled over. Friends called and I didn't want to talk to them. I was angry at all of them for being healthy, being carefree. But I knew that carefree state of being could change instantly for any of us—on a dime, as the saying goes. Nothing had ever felt truer than that phrase.

I focused on the next day's news stories. Former U.S. President Bill Clinton had just been diagnosed with four-vessel disease and undergone bypass surgery. Local radio stations had been calling to get a clip from me about his condition. The CTV nightly news, however, decided they didn't want a talk-back on Clinton; I was not needed. They would report the story without a medical commentary. They were concerned that this was too American a story and did not require my medical input. I shook my head in disbelief. *Heart disease is the number-one killer of North Americans. Maybe we should go to air with wait times for surgery in Canada. That is truly a Canadian story.* I laughed at how my anger was filtering even the medical news. Waiting times had been one of the key issues of the recent Canadian election. And while it was a great issue for elections, wait times are still horrendous in Canada. Bill Clinton didn't have to wait four weeks to get his surgery. I did. Even with my medical connections, I was waiting. The emotional toll of that wait is impossible to measure. I empathize daily with my patients about wait times; I understand their anger. I am constantly on the phone arbitrating on their behalf to get those tests, referrals, results. That is why my patients are so loyal. They know that I will push for them as best I can in a system that is so bogged down.

I was living the system. I understood it, but it didn't help my anger. I understood that priorities dictate test times and surgical times, but I was left wondering how much cancer you must have to get treatment faster. I knew my surgeon was booked and that getting me in earlier would mean cancelling someone else who likely had waited longer than me. The rational Marla got this. The irrational, angry Marla did not. *Nine more days. Nine more days for my malignant cells to multiply, spread, invade.* Those cells were not my friends.

We were scheduled to leave for Florida at the end of the week for a girlfriend's 50th birthday party, but I had decided not to go. I sat down with my girlfriend and explained why I could not come. She was supportive, and horrified for me, but I warned her not to feel sorry for me. I felt sorry enough for myself. She reminded me I was indestructible. I wished I could believe her. The next day, Tuesday, was an intimate dinner with six very close friends to celebrate her birthday. I had warned them that my so-called illness was not to be a topic for conversation. I had also told them that if anyone made a toast to good health, I would get up and walk away. If anyone made a toast to friendship, I would walk away. I could imagine them all rolling their eyes at my ridiculous demands, but they were willing to humour me. I was torn about going at all, but most of me felt that I did want to go and be among those good friends. Staying home and pitying myself didn't seem to be helping a whole lot. I promised I would go.

I found myself smiling, remembering a moment with these friends during the summer. Every summer we go away—a total of eight of us—to one couple's cottage for a weekend full of great food, incredible friendship, silly behaviour and a whole lot of wine. We had been there just a few weeks ago while all the kids were away at camp. One afternoon, when the guys had gone golfing, the four of us lay on the dock sharing what we call dock talk. I have spent countless days and hours on that dock. With this group I have shared much—my pregnancy losses, my pregnancy attempts. It was there that I went after Jason died. Every summer I write a silly poem about our weekend in the guest book. The summer he died was the only summer I didn't write a poem. Instead I wrote a heartfelt letter about the nurturing of friendships. This most recent summer afternoon was hot, and we had dispensed with our bathing-suit tops. We were joking about my picture showing up in the *National Enquirer* when the golfers returned a little earlier than expected. The men were stunned by the sight of the four of us, and we laughed hysterically. Now I found myself wondering what I would look like next summer and if I would be as liberal with my bathing-suit top. As odd as the visual imagery was, it made me smile: *I know these friends will take me as I come.*

Tuesday was the first day back at work after the Labour Day weekend. One of my patients, whom I have cared for over many years, had just found out that her breast cancer had spread to her liver. She needed to see me. As much as I didn't want to do this, I knew I had to—my personal life has no place in my professional life. We sat and talked for an hour. She was frightened, and rightfully so. We went over her options. She wanted to talk about alternative medicine, experimental procedures in Europe and Argentina. I listened and reviewed what was known and what was not. I could now understand, on a totally different level, her need to take control and go where there was no evidence of benefit. It had been 10 years since her diagnosis. Chemotherapy had failed her. Evidence-based medicine had failed her. She knew there was no longer a cure, only time, and that the clock was ticking faster. I put her in touch with some leading researchers but I knew this was time for her. I hoped we could control and ultimately palliate, but we could not cure. I was as supportive of her as I could be, not once allowing myself to lose sight of what I was doing. It was hard. My secretary looked at me knowingly when the patient left. I kept going through the day, pushing what was happening to me deep below the surface.

I found the time to track down Dr. Karina Bukhanov, following up on her voicemail over the weekend about the lesion on my left breast. She told me that the lesion was visible in the progressive phase of the MRI. I had misunderstood her earlier use of the word *progressive*: it was not the lesion that was progressive. It appeared benign to her but she could not guarantee it. It was not possible to do the same kind of localization under an MRI that could be done with an ultrasound or mammography. The metal hook could not be used in an MRI because of the magnetic resonators: metal causes a lot of shimmer and distortion on the films. There was a tool available but it was not available in Toronto. "Where is it?" I ranted. "Why can't it be sent? I will gladly pay for it." She was sympathetic but told me it wouldn't be here for at least a week and she would be in Seattle the following week—the week that I was scheduled for surgery.

While I tried hard not to slay the messenger—Karina has been so helpful and empathetic—I was furious. I was beginning to realize that both breasts would not be treated at the same time, and so I shifted my focus to deal again with the disease I knew about: the right breast, the malignant breast. I wondered aloud if David had had any cancellations, and if my surgery could therefore be moved up. Karina told me she would speak to David about it. She told me that the next day would be my final MRI, to do a single of the right breast, my diseased, cancerous breast. We hung up, but shortly afterwards she called to say that Dr. McCready could push up the surgery to the day after tomorrow, Thursday, September 9.

I was ecstatic that at least the right breast would be operated on soon. But I was afraid I had misheard. I knew how tight David's schedule was, and I knew that he would not cancel someone else's surgery to make time for me. Neither of us could do that. I asked my secretary to call his office and confirm that I had heard right. We got his voicemail, but within the hour his secretary called back: he did have the OR time but I would be the last case of the day. I couldn't have cared less. It was going to happen. I told my office staff to cancel Thursday and I reminded them that this was to be kept quiet.

At home, I got ready to go out for my friend's birthday dinner. I was relieved that the surgery was now 48 hours away, but I would not talk about it at dinner. I had decided to tell no one. Bobby and I talked about plausible reasons to explain our not going to Florida. Hurricane Frances was ripping through Florida, affording me with an excuse. I watched the devastation on the television screen and thought how much it felt like what was going on inside me. I reminded myself that I was not without options and to toughen up a little and not be so self-indulgent. We then decided that since I had told CTV about my negotiations with ABC, we would tell everyone that I had to go back for more talks. It would give them something good to talk about.

Rolling through my head were some conversations with friends over the past few days, some of whom would be at this dinner. I am often invited to speak about finding balance, and in that presentation I talk about decision-making, about going to your "board of directors." We all have a board of directors. They are that group of women and men you feel closest to, who can listen to you, put aside their own agendas and advise you as friends. You are fortunate if you can identify one or two women who can do that for you. In my case, I was—and am—lucky enough to have several women. But even with these women, I knew they could not put aside their personal agenda of wanting me to be well and healthy. Every time they offered me reassurances, I reminded them that none of us really knows. Their assurances somehow made me angrier because we just didn't know. Mercifully, they put up with my ranting. They knew I was crazed. I was also the only one of my age group with a nine-year-old.

They all knew what I was thinking. I couldn't help going there, as much as they tried to derail that kind of thinking; as much as I yelled at myself for being self-indulgent, those thoughts kept creeping in. I promised myself to try to push them away. There was no place for negative thinking. I tried to make that my mantra. *Tomorrow is another day. These truisms—where the hell do they come from? Then again, they have some validity. Okay,* I told myself, *tomorrow is another day and it brings me one day closer to surgery. One day closer to some answers, as awful as those answers might be.* I have always told my patients that knowledge empowers you, and I truly believe it. I believed that once I had a game plan, I would feel more in control. Everything felt out of my control right then. I reminded myself that my feelings were normal. I would have to do better at dealing with uncertainty. But for this one night, at a birthday celebration, I did not want to go through those conversations again. I wanted someone else to be the focus of conversation.

The next day was September 8, and Susan and Renee, two of my girlfriends, insisted on taking me down for the last MRI. Karina came in to talk to me while I climbed up on the table. The familiar intravenous line was started. My arms were getting bruised. Carol, the head technician, and I had become good friends by now. We talked about the left breast, and they pointed out that the left-side lesion was on the medial, or inside, aspect of the left breast. I immediately understood the technical difficulties of getting an accurate picture: the patient lies face down, the two breasts hanging through the openings, with the right breast in the way of the left breast. I pointed out that I am small, and suggested that I scoot the left breast into the right hole and contort myself into a pretzel for a better chance at a clear image. They had also been thinking of this—the night before, Karina (who is about the same size as me) had actually attempted the awkward position. She told me it was hard and I would have to hold that position for an hour. But I was highly motivated, and so we decided that after we completed the MRI on the right side we would do a test run.

When the time came, I carefully positioned myself. They covered my head with a pillowcase and slowly inched me into the machine. I felt my right shoulder butt up against the machine wall, but I was in position. They got me back out and asked me if I could withstand that for an hour. Piece of cake, I told them. But despite the fact that we had conquered the difficulty of getting at the site, the tool was still not yet available, and therefore the biopsy of the left breast could not be done in time for the next day's surgery. I was angry, but knew that I was behaving like a petulant child. Karina had done so much for me, moving up the MRIs and fitting me into cancellations and rare holes in the schedule. Tomorrow I would be in at 9 a.m. for the needle localization on the right and then the injections to find the nodes, but Karina would not be at Princess Margaret for that. I gave both Carol and Karina a hug, thanked them for everything, and choked back tears as I said goodbye.

I changed and got ready to leave. Susan and Renee were waiting. Karina came out and said goodbye and told me she would see me the next day. (So she would be coming by to oversee the procedure after all!) Both my friends asked why. I told them it was just another "look-see." I had not told them about the surgery.

We went downstairs and I said goodbye to Susan. She was leaving for Florida in the morning, although she was anxious about the impending hurricane. I told her not to be angry, knowing she would be furious that I had not shared the OR date with her. She looked at me quizzically as she got into her car.

Renee and I navigated the traffic to North York General Hospital at the other end of town. I am on staff at several hospitals. I had arranged to have my genetic testing done there for the three most common gene mutations that I am likely to have as an Ashkenazi Jew. People of Ashkenazi Jewish ancestry run a higher than usual risk of having three particular gene mutations that can lead to inherited forms of breast cancer. I do not have a family history of breast or ovarian cancer, but if I proved gene-positive then I would elect to remove both breasts.

Renee looked at me in the car and asked me what Karina had meant. I told her about the surgery. But she had already figured it out.

We got to the hospital and Dr. Wendy Meschino, a geneticist and colleague who has appeared on my show, was waiting for me. Renee came in with me and Dr. Meschino treated me like any other patient. She explained the common mutations that we are aware of. More genetic testing is available but she was not recommending it. She felt that these three were the most critical for me. We agreed. She confirmed that I understood what positive findings would mean. I reassured her that I had done this counselling many times for many other patients. I told her that it meant I would have my breasts and uterus removed if the results were positive. I told her that I could indeed give her informed consent. I discussed what the test results would mean for my children. If I was gene positive, then it meant there was a chance my children would be positive as well. I would have to face the possibility that they could inherit the gene from me and an increased risk of cancer as well. The thought was frightening. With all that discussed I went upstairs to have my blood drawn.

The technician was delighted to see me. She told me her husband loved me and the show and she could not wait to tell him she had seen me. I interrupted her gently, reminding her that this would be a breach of confidentiality. She said she was nervous about drawing my blood. In an attempt to reassure her I told her I have great veins—despite the fact that my veins are small and difficult to get a sample from. While she was prepping I suggested that she tell her husband she had bumped into me in the halls and we chatted, and asked her to thank him for me for watching the show. With that, a long day at best, Renee and I headed home. I was emotionally exhausted.

Renee and I got home and shut the door to my office and discussed what would happen the next day. The phone rang, but I ignored it; I was picking up messages on my cellphone. David's secretary had called to confirm the OR time. When I picked up the messages on my home phone, there was one from Karina. She told me to come in at 7 a.m. so that she and Carol could attempt the MRI localization of the left breast after all. It would be with the wrong tool, but she was prepared if I was prepared. We were about to make history.

We ate dinner. None of this felt real at all. Renee told me she would be over at six in the morning to get me. Bobby would drive in his own car.

I could hardly sleep at all, I was so anxious for the morning to come. I told Amanda and Matt I was going to New York again, which I had done during the summer for the ABC talks. They thought nothing of it. Finally it was 5:30 a.m. and, having watched each hour pass on the clock, I got up. I kissed each of the kids as they slept, then left.

I arrived at the MRI unit and was greeted by a patient of mine who was there for a knee MRI. Bobby and Renee were horrified for me but I couldn't have cared less. He probably thought I was there for the same reason, I told them.

Karina and Carol positioned me as we had planned: left breast in the right breast opening and the rest of my body contorted so that I could be slid into the MRI scanner. Again an IV was started. The first 30 minutes were devoted to scanning to localize the suspicious area. I was told they had practised on a grapefruit and, though there was splay and distortion in the MRI images, they felt fairly confident that, once the needle was inserted into the breast and it was rescanned, Dr. Bukhanov would be able to accurately place the needle into the area in question. I was game. I was quiet and cooperative. To attempt this with the tools that were available was the only choice I had.

After 30 minutes they slid me out. The entire time my left breast had been placed in a clamp so that it would not move. While this had not been done with the other MRIs, it had to be done in this case so the breast wouldn't move when the radiologist attempted to insert the hook. I was face down and could not see anything. Karina was ready, crouching below the table to place the hook in. She warned me: "Needle poke." A small wire with a sleeve pierced my skin, and though it hurt I did not flinch. They slid me back into the machine to see if Karina had placed it in the right area. She had done this based on the "map" in her head, translated from the MRI images, of where she should go. I realized how technically difficult this was for her. They slid me back out: she had to readjust the hook.

I knew it would hurt as she pushed it deeper and more laterally. I did not move or say a word. Karina asked me if I was okay and I assured her I was indeed fine. They slid me one more time back into the MRI machine: she was now happy with the placement. I was slid back out. Karina and Carol got me up gently; they didn't want me to inadvertently move the hook. They withdrew the sleeve that covered the hook and its arms opened and became anchored in my breast. They taped down the wire hanging out of my breast. It had been uncomfortable, but by no means intolerable.

They told me I was incredible, but I replied that they were the incredible ones. I was overwhelmed at the lengths they had gone to make this happen for me, and so very grateful. I told them that I was the best patient to have attempted this on because I could truly give informed consent. Relief washed over me: at last I would have an answer as to what was in that breast, my so-called healthy left breast.

Bobby, Renee and I walked down the connecting corridor

to Princess Margaret Hospital, next door to Mount Sinai. I looked down at the floor as I walked, not wanting to see anyone I knew. We checked in to the 18th floor, where I was kindly ushered into a small room, since my room wasn't ready. The staff, knowing that I was a familiar face in the hospital because of being on air and being on staff at these institutions, were trying to protect my anonymity, trying to let me be just a patient. Anyone there would know this was an outpatient surgical floor. It would be clear why I was there.

At 9 a.m. we took my chart and went down to the third floor. Dr. Bukhanov was there, just as she had promised. She told me she wanted to do the right breast localization under ultrasound. Again, because we could not feel the tumour, only visualize it under imagery, the surgeon would need a map as to where to operate. These localizations would tell him where the tumour was. It is the same principle as the core biopsies, but done without any freezing. Karina did the ultrasound but had trouble finding the area. I had had a menstrual cycle since the initial ultrasound and everything now looked different. She found an area she did not like. She sent in the wire and told me my breasts were like cement they were so dense. She was having trouble placing the wire. I told her to go ahead and push. She knew this was unpleasant at best. I was holding my breath. She re-examined me with the ultrasound but was not happy with the placement and decided to do another. I told her this was fine, she was not to worry: I wanted her to be completely happy with the placement, and accurate. *I have cancer. I am highly motivated. I ignore the pain.* She inserted another wire and told me again how tough my breasts were. I attempted to laugh and reminded her that nothing is straightforward with me.

Then we walked over to mammography to see if the hooks were in the right place. My breast was tender and the thought of having it compressed in a mammogram machine wasn't appealing. When Karina looked at the finished films, she was not happy and called David from the OR. He looked and told her he wanted another wire. I held my breath. They decided the best way to do this was to repeat the set-up they had used with the stereotactic core. My breast was held in place by two clamps, the x-ray localized the area of calcifications and another wire was put in place. A final mammogram was done.

A nurse was holding me upright; she thought I was going to pass out. I knew this was not the norm and that technically my case was difficult, but I was not going to pass out. I came out of the procedure walking but feeling nauseated. I was pale. I was grateful. They reminded me that usually this takes only one pass-through with a wire, but my breasts were dense and the tumour would not declare itself. In surgery, David McCready would need clear dimensions as to where to begin and end, and so this had all been necessary. I understood all this, and was grateful—thrilled, in fact—that this part was behind me. David asked me if I was getting any radio signals yet, I had so many wires. I tried to laugh. Renee and Bobby were both stunned at what I had been through, but I was not. I was grateful for the technology and expertise that had gotten me there.

I asked if the next part would be any easier. Both David and Karina told me honestly: no, the next part would be painful. Now *I* was stunned. How could it get more difficult? But I was halfway there. I was so relieved to be getting on with this. Together, the three of us headed back to Mount Sinai's nuclear medicine department.

I was about to undergo a somewhat new procedure called

sentinel node removal. Instead of removing all the lymph nodes, which was likely not necessary, this procedure would identify those nodes that drained the tumour, since those are the nodes most likely to show cancer if the cancer had spread. Cancer doesn't play hopscotch but moves along through the drainage system in an orderly fashion. The challenge would be to find the nodes that were the drainers of my cancer, and remove them during surgery later in the day.

David spoke to the radiologist about where he wanted him to inject me. The radiologist, Dr. Marlon Hershkop, explained that he would inject a nuclear tracer four times directly into my breast, infiltrating the cancerous area. We would watch under a scanner where the tracer went, that is, where the radioactivity was. The lymph nodes that drained this area would pick up the radioactive tracer, and with a Geiger counter David could find them and remove them at the time of surgery. The technology was fascinating—despite what this meant to me personally, I was curious and astounded at what medicine could do. David said the good news was that removing only the affected lymph nodes meant I would likely not run into complications of arm swelling and lymphedema. The bad news was that the procedure was painful. With all these warnings, I began to wonder just how painful it would be.

I lay down on the table to begin, but the soreness in my breast made it hard to lift my arms over my head. I finally found a position I could tolerate. Dr. Hershkop told me that it would feel like bee stings. I held my breath as he injected directly into my right breast, near the nipple area. As the radioactive particles were injected, I knew that he was right: it felt like one long bee sting. I braced myself for three more injections, but aside from the occasional gasp and saying "Yikes," I didn't flinch. I could think of better ways to spend my day but, once again, my relief at moving along was stronger than the pain.

Then we waited. The tracer needed time to pool and travel to my nodes. On the screen we could see the radioactive material pooling, the four shots coalescing into one large pool of radioactive material. As time marched on we could see the material move into the right armpit. Lymph nodes seemed to light up. It was impossible to tell if it was one or two. I was hoping for two or three normal nodes so I could be confident. I was willing them to be normal.

The radiologist took a radioactive pencil and actually outlined my body like an Etch-a-Sketch. The outline of my body showed up on the screen. It was fascinating. Still using the radioactive pencil, he continued marking my body, and watched as his markings matched up with where the lymph nodes were showing on the screen. He marked an area under my armpit with a permanent marker, the same kind of marker I use to mark my kids' clothes when they are going to camp. This was not camp. He placed an X so David would know where to make his incision into my armpit. I was ready for surgery.

We walked back to Princess Margaret. I crawled into bed and found a position I could tolerate. Renee picked up her cellphone messages and found that Susan had called: she hadn't gone to Florida after all. She offloaded her bags when they got news that the hurricane was heading towards Key West. She had left messages on my cell and Renee's cell. She had attempted to find Bobby. She knew something was up.

Renee called Susan and filled her in. Before Renee could hang up, Susan was in her car. I knew that Anne, my other dear friend, would be furious with me, but she was giving her niece a bridal shower and I could not see the point in alarming her. The hospital room phone rang. We all looked startled. It was my doctor and friend, Vivien. She had received a faxed notification of my admission and had tracked me down.

The system is seldom this efficient—just my luck it actually was this time. I filled her in but I was having a hard time talking. I didn't want her to be mad at me. I didn't want anyone to be mad at me. I just wanted to keep moving forward as quietly as possible. I didn't want to offend anyone, but I had to do it this way.

And then Bobby's cellphone rang. It was my sister-in-law Wendy. She and I had both been scheduled for surgical procedures on the same day a week from now. She had a benign lesion that she had been advised to remove. The secretary called to confirm her procedure and told her she was moving her up into my time. When asked why, the secretary told her I was having surgery now, today. Wendy panicked. What could have happened to make them move up the surgery? Bobby filled her in. Seems there is no confidentiality. My intention was not to alarm anyone but it seemed to have been unavoidable.

I had told my sister about the surgery but she has difficulty flying and decided she could not come. She was devastated, and I was disappointed. My anger at everything spilled over at her. I wanted her to come. I knew she could not. I had to understand.

All I wanted now was to be left alone and go for surgery. We waited.

As we waited, the dietitian stuck in her head to ask me if I had any dietary restrictions. We reminded her I was NPO—nothing by mouth—before surgery. She wanted to know about dinner that night. Renee laughed at the question of dietary restrictions and quipped, "She eats everything—but no carbs, pasta or rice, nothing white or fried, must be fat-free, nothing with sauce or dressing . . ." I started to laugh at how ludicrous this all was. The dietitian made a hasty retreat.

Finally the orderly came to get me. My procession now included Bobby, Renee and Susan. Wendy Freeman, the executive producer of the CTV *National News,* had left voicemail messages. She was the only one at the network who knew about my diagnosis and had promised to protect my confidentiality. I was grateful. She left a message that she couldn't find me and, with a nose for news—journalist that she is—she was suspicious. She knew I had wanted to move things along and now she thought she had cracked this story. I smiled—as always, she was right. We had talked about the fact that I would have to go public eventually. I jokingly promised that when I did I would give her the exclusive. She laughed at me. I wanted to go public, particularly if it was helpful, much in the same way we did with Jason. But I had to do it when I was ready. Wendy understood.

We headed down to surgery and I was the last case of the day. I am latex-allergic and the OR had to be completely prepped to be latex-free. The orderly had everyone come into pre-op with me, where David had my films up on the computer. He was studying them and I was busy telling him what to do. I asked how much he planned to take, and told him—not for the first time—to take more rather than less. I assured him that my days as a stripper were over. I knew I must be trying his patience but he smiled and endured my directions. I told him not to worry: soon he could call in the anesthetist to shut me up.

David told me that he had decided to do a frozen section of the sentinel nodes since he would have time. What this means is that while I was asleep, the nodes would be removed and "flash-frozen" and the pathologist would look to see if there was any cancer. If there were signs of cancer, David would remove more than just the sentinel nodes. Originally his plan was to operate on only one breast but now he would be operating on both. He would start on the right side, and while he moved over to the left side, the pathologist would have ample time to prepare a frozen section. He told me that if I woke up with a drain it would mean the node was positive and he had done a complete dissection. I re-signed the consent form, allowing him to do this if necessary. Bobby gave me a kiss. I flashed everyone one last look at my "before" breasts. They wheeled me in. Showtime . . . live . . . there was no time for retakes.

I was placed on the table in the quintessential white-and-green operating room, a room made familiar by countless television shows and, in my case, my training. The nurse was kind as she wrapped me in a warm blanket and placed a pillow under my knees and a mask over my face. In a minute, I knew, I would be out cold. They warned me about a one-in-a-thousand risk of a broken tooth. I nodded and suddenly I could hear a voice in my head asking for more time, for a way out. Maybe all this was just a nightmare. Maybe the disease really would be early, non-invasive. Yup, Kübler-Ross was right: there are stages and here I was, bargaining. I could feel myself drifting.

And the next thing I knew it was the recovery room. I could feel myself groping towards my right armpit. The nurse came over to me, and I asked her if I had a drain. She looked a little confused but told me no, I did not have a drain. I knew then that my sentinels were negative, and I was grateful, cautiously grateful. Bobby entered the room and was relieved to see me. I told him I didn't have a drain but I felt really nauseated. He was just happy to see me.

I was wheeled back up to the room on the 18th floor. I had been given morphine, which made me itchy. I was groggy but fighting sleep. Bobby and I decided to call Amanda and Jenna. Amanda cried. I told her to take a cab and come to the hospital and see that I was really fine. It seemed that she arrived in a matter of moments. I had lost my timeline.

I called Jenna, who was away at school. She started to cry. I felt so bad to put them through this. They had already been through so much in their young lives. She was angry at me but I told her this was all last-minute, that the schedule changed and Dr. McCready could fit me in. It was her first day of school. What was the point of worrying her? It was over, and I was fine. Still, she was upset to be so far away. I asked her whom she felt closest to. I asked her if she thought she could trust them to protect my request to keep this quiet, at least until I knew everything and my parents knew. I told her to go to her friends, confide in them. I know the value of a good cry and a hug. I know the value of the friends who are standing by me.

I also knew that my larger community of friends, others who would have liked to know about my surgery, would be upset. It was not that I wanted to keep this a secret over the long term. It was not even that I had chosen those friends I trust more or care for more. I was simply trying to protect myself, for now, from their sympathetic looks, their wishes for my health that tended to make me feel angry instead of consoled. And—more important—I was waiting until I had more answers for myself. I needed answers desperately, for myself first and foremost. Everything that I balance felt so precarious at that time. How could I make plans when everything was out of my control? I needed to have a plan before I could tell my parents. My friends call me a control freak. It's true that I am organized; you have to be to do everything I do. And I had learned the lesson that so much in life is out of our control. I was relearning that lesson.

Jenna knew I wanted to keep this confidential and she was reluctant to go to a friend, but I insisted. She told me she would, and assured me she would call later. Amanda arrived just as I said goodbye to her sister. She started to cry but seemed happy to be there. I asked her to call Jenna and reassure her that I was fine. *I am fine. I am relieved to have this part over.*

Now the next round of waiting began. It felt as though I would be waiting for the rest of my life . . . waiting for results, waiting to see if I recurred over time. Yet I refused to live my life in suspension. I had just given an interview about the new season of *Balance*. I remembered what I had said: "Don't feel consumed by what you do. Find the time to invest in the things that make you happy. Make sure that you are living life as opposed to life living you." The so-called good doctor was trying to remember her own advice.

It was time for everyone to leave the hospital. Finally I was alone with my thoughts and my fears. I made it through the night. There had not been an order for sleep medication, and I was amazed by my extreme fatigue yet my total inability to sleep. Surprisingly, the pain was not bad at all. I was uncomfortable but the pain was entirely tolerable, though I had not taken any medication. I was willing it to be morning but it took a long time to finally see six o'clock. I called Bobby in his car. I had asked him to go to work; my sister-in-law Wendy would be coming to get me. Vivien, my friend and doctor, dropped by my room, and I knew she must have come down extra early to see me before going to her office. She brought me yogurt. We were both glad that I was on this side of the surgery. I couldn't wait to be home.

Wendy got there shortly after Viv left. We were waiting for the resident to come in and discharge me. When the resident arrived, I asked questions about the extra stitches on the left breast. They were placed there because of bleeding and I was told that I could remove them in five days. She confirmed that I could take a shower in two days and remove the dressings at that time. I was not to exercise or exert. I should not work for a week. I was committed to do *Canada AM* Monday and Tuesday but I agreed that I would not go to the office. I didn't think of half a day on Tuesday as a real day—I fail to mention that.

We gathered my things and headed home. I felt a little light-headed as we walked outside to the car, but I was so happy to be going home.

I fell into my bed at home and finally fell asleep for three hours. I asked my housekeeper to simply say I was unavailable if anyone called. I had not told her what was going on.

Matt got home after school. He wanted to know if I was sick or simply not feeling well. I am not sure what the difference was in his young mind but I told him I was not feeling well. He seemed happy with that answer. He plunked himself down in my room to do his homework, and seemed unperturbed that I was in bed and my girlfriends were over. Believe me, this was unusual, but Matt just rolled with it.

Amanda arrived home, upset. Her girlfriend's dad had suddenly passed away and she was planning to go to the viewing that evening. We talked about it and later she headed off. But when she came home, she fell apart on my bed. She cried as she talked about her friend's dad not being at her friend's graduation, her friend's wedding. These thoughts had echoed in my own mind and I knew she was thinking about us as well. These were my fears and thoughts every time I looked at my own children—particularly when I looked at Matt. We talked about how unfair life can be. She told me that she knew there was nothing she could say to her girlfriend to comfort her. She was right. I told my very wise 17-year-old that she knew more than most adults. Most people make stupid, trite comments. There are no words to make the pain go away, I agreed, but what she could do as a friend was be there to support her, even if it was just to listen or take her for a drive. Just be there.

It as much as anyone can do. I remembered some of the stupid things people said during the period after Jason's death. I think in part that is why I had been so private about this frightening bout of cancer: it helped me avoid some of the ridiculous comments that are meant to be helpful but are exactly the opposite. Amanda fell asleep in my bed and I reminded myself, *I still have a lot to do. I am not ready to go anywhere. I need to be here for my kids. I need them as much as they need me.*

FIVE

Breast cancer won't kill me, anxiety will

Saturday, and I was lying around, preparing some work for *Canada AM* on the Monday. I took a shower and washed my hair, struggling but managing to get that right arm up. I removed the dressings, leaving the Steri-strips—sterile adhesive bandages for closing surgical wounds—holding the incisions together. For the first time I could see clearly what Dr. McCready had done, including the neat horizontal incisions on each breast. There was a lot of swelling under the right arm; it felt like a tennis ball was stuck there. With so much swelling it was impossible to know what my breasts would look like later, but I couldn't care less.

That night, Anne, Susan, Renee and their husbands joined us at home for dinner, with lots of wine. I showed my girlfriends my incisions, and they were impressed. I was impressed. My badges of honour. But I was wondering—what was around the corner? Yet these women and I had been friends forever. They helped me relax and have a good time, and I was not focused every minute on my cancer.

On Sunday, I awoke to incredible burning in both breasts and the armpit. Bobby had left early for Chicago on business. I looked down and saw a terrible rash peeking out from under the Steri-strips. I was clearly having an allergic reaction to the adhesive. I am latex-allergic and the adhesive must have been latex-based. My skin was swollen and pustular. I could not believe it. This felt entirely unfair.

I tried to track down Vivien and a friend who is a dermatologist, but no one was around. I paged the surgical resident and we both agreed the Steri-strips had to be removed.

Amanda was home, and I asked her if she was up for helping me with this. Even as I asked, I was thinking, *No child should have to do this for her mother.* But she said she could do it, and together we removed the strips from each breast and the right armpit. Part of the nipple on the left side was not sewn down and it lifted up as the strips were removed. We were both shocked. I was horrified for Amanda but she was steady and calm.

I called in a prescription for cortisone and a topical antibiotic. We applied it and waited for it to have an effect, but I was not a happy camper. Wendy Freeman stopped by on her way home from the newsroom, where their focus was the hurricane ravaging the United States. She asked me the obvious: why had I not called my own doctor? Even though patients manage to track me down and call me at home all the time, I was reluctant to do the same. Wendy yelled at me, and I was able to find Dr. McCready's phone number. I managed to catch him at home—ironically, just before he headed out to help with the Walk to End Breast Cancer for Princess Margaret Hospital. When I described what had happened, he told me to put on dry dressings, then leave it alone and come and see him in the morning.

I was relieved. This was another reminder that I was the patient in this situation and I didn't have to solve these problems myself. But the patient role is tough for me, not to my liking, and not a role that I'm good at. What seemed obvious to Wendy simply did not occur to me.

I was glad to be seeing David the next day; it would give me a chance to ask him what he had done during the surgery. I knew he had spoken to me after the surgery but I could not recall a word. In the meantime, I tried to ignore how irritating this damn rash was. I was going to ice it until tomorrow. Tomorrow. It seemed I was always waiting for tomorrow.

On Monday morning I was out of bed at five. I sensed that the rash was worse but I didn't want to look at it. I got dressed in the dark and headed out to find the CTV driver waiting for me. This morning on *Canada AM* I would be offering commentary on the upcoming health care talks in Ottawa, where the main focus was on shortening wait times for treatment of all kinds. As a physician I understand the frustration of my patients, who can wait months for elective MRIs, or up to a year and a half for knee and hip replacement surgeries. I was living this frustration myself now, and I knew that my time from diagnosis to surgery had been abbreviated by my being my own advocate and not having had to wait to see intervening physicians.

I was on air with Michael Decter, a health care policy consultant, and we talked about the severe national shortage of technology, physicians, nurses and pharmacists. We talked about the inadequate numbers in medical school, the numbers of physicians leaving. With a shudder I thought about the possibility of Dr. McCready leaving one day. We had recently lost one of our star oncologists from Princess Margaret to Massachusetts General in the U.S. Michael Decter observed that Canada's stars, be they actors or doctors, often get lured to their version of Hollywood. The comment was not lost on me as I thought of my talks with ABC.

Before we knew it, the segment was done and I was heading down to Princess Margaret to see David. I looked pretty good for someone post-op—but then, everyone does when the masters of makeup at CTV make them camera-ready. I was ushered into an examining room where Dr. McCready's nurse helped me take off my suit. We both gasped when we saw the angry mess my right armpit was. My breasts hadn't fared much better. I was a disaster.

Dr. McCready came in, took a look and sympathetically agreed: this was awful. He had seen reactions to tape before, he said, but never like this. Of course, ever the overachiever, I have to excel even at getting rashes and allergic reactions. I apologized to David for having called him at home, but he brushed it off. The problem now was not only the allergic reaction, but also the fact that without the Steri-strips to hold everything in place my healing was somewhat compromised. The last thing we wanted was a secondary infection. He was adamant that I not see patients and suggested that I keep the area dry, apply nothing at all and start an antibiotic. He prescribed a 10-day course of a broad-spectrum antibiotic. As far as I knew I was not allergic. We looked at each other and hoped I was right.

I asked if he could tell me again how the surgery had gone. He told me that he had removed three lymph nodes, even though the third had very little radioactivity in it and likely could have been left. He had respected my wish to err on the side of aggression while not compromising his decision-making. The two active nodes, when analyzed by frozen section during the operation, had been found negative, and he had closed the incision in the armpit. On the right side, where the tumour had been ("had been"—that sounded good), he removed a generous portion of tissue. The removal of tissue on the left breast, my so-called healthy side, was dictated by the placement of the hook during the MRI localization. However, when he went to close the incision in the right breast, the breast with the known cancer, he felt an area that was somewhat firmer around where the hooks were and, respecting my wishes to err on the side of aggression, he removed that as well.

I asked David when I should see him again. Knowing that I would likely pester the pathologists for results, he told me to call him when the pathology report was ready. As protective as I am of my own patients, always calling for their results, I would almost certainly do the same for myself. Dr. McCready was used to my behaviour as a doctor, and he must have known that I could not leave that role behind and simply be a patient. Being a patient, I realized again, was hard and unfamiliar work. I knew that the pathology report was likely to be ready at the end of the week, and we arranged for Dr. McCready's secretary to call me and book an appointment.

I got home and could not imagine what I would do with myself for the remainder of the week. I am used to juggling many jobs, but sitting at home is not one of them. I read every embargoed medical story for the upcoming week, sent dozens of e-mails and prepared stories for the next day's show. My e-mails must have been driving everyone else crazy.

I kept trying to anticipate what the next few weeks would be like, what I might have to cancel if I had to do radiation or more surgery. Control, control: I reminded myself that I had limited control in this mass of chaos. I had to let go. Maybe my television focus should shift from medical reporting to soap operas. My life was beginning to feel like one.

Despite following my doctor's orders, the rash got worse. Over the next two days, it continued to burn and itch and weep, worse even than before. I was beside myself. I could hardly cope with the ridiculousness of this unanticipated side effect, and with the thought that if it didn't clear up and I needed radiation, the rash would cause a delay. I called Dr. Gordon Sussman, the allergist and immunologist who cared for me when I was first diagnosed with a latex allergy. He asked me to come to his office but at that point I felt so ill I could not manage the drive. He lives close to me and offered to stop in after work. I was incredibly grateful.

Late in the afternoon he arrived to confirm that this was a dreadful case of contact dermatitis. He was sorry for me— the breast cancer, and now this whole mess. He told me what I already suspected, that I needed high-dose prednisone; a topical cream wouldn't touch this rash, and if we didn't get it under control it could affect my whole body. I knew he was right and, though I was aware of the possible side effects, I agreed to start a whopping dose of prednisone, plus a medication to protect my stomach from ulcers. We agreed to stop the antibiotic since I didn't really need it. The swelling under my arm was so severe that I couldn't get dressed or put my arm down. I was angry, furious even. I knew this was all unanticipated, yet I felt as though my body had let me down again. It felt endless.

The next day I had a meeting with Robert Hurst, the president of network news at CTV. I had arranged this meeting some time before, and I wanted to use it to discuss where I was going at CTV and to talk about my frustrations. He is a busy man but he fit me into his schedule. He was aware of the contract offer from ABC and in his own distinguished career had worked both sides of the border and all over the globe. I was anxious to talk to him, and determined to make the meeting. He had no clue about my health issues.

I sat through the meeting trying to ignore the way I felt. We talked about my roles—both current and potential—at the network, whether I had perceived value and what the American offer meant. He was honest with me, at times critical, but listened to my issues carefully. He told me he would speak with *Canada AM* and *National News* and get back to me. I could not believe that I had seriously been considering ABC. If ever a wake-up call had been given, breast cancer certainly had woken me up. The American offer would have meant weekly travel and limited holiday time. The lure of moving my career forward had become irrelevant. I wanted to be with my family—that much was clearer to me than ever. And maybe it was enough just to be invited to the party. Maybe I didn't need to go to the party. It had been enough just to be considered for the job.

It was the night before Rosh Hashanah, the Jewish New Year, and traditionally a family night. We were expected the next day at a luncheon and, later in the day, for a large family dinner at my mother-in-law's. For tonight, though, the first night, our own family would dine together, just the five of us—even Jenna, who would be home from university—and I was determined to make this a special night.

I pulled out all the stops to make a huge dinner and tried to immerse myself totally in the cooking and baking, preparing enough for an army. I made each of the kids' favourite cakes. The house smelled good but I was still anxious and finding it hard to stay in the moment.

Finally, I picked up the phone and called pathology at Princess Margaret Hospital. I spoke to the pathologist, which was somewhat ludicrous, given that I was the patient. But I spoke to these people on a regular basis about my patients and I could not force myself just to sit back. I realized how uncomfortable this was for these consultants, who don't, as a rule, speak to patients much; they communicate with other doctors, not doctor-patients. I didn't care.

The pathologist somewhat curtly reminded me that my breast tissue and lymph nodes were still radioactive, having been injected pre-operatively to locate the sentinel nodes. While the surgery had freed me of the radioactivity and I had urinated out the rest, that in the breast specimen (as she called it) had to decay naturally over time. That of course meant it had to sit for several days before it could be prepared to be read. I told her not to rush anything and to treat this like anyone else's tissue. I felt entirely stupid. I thanked her but knew it would be at least another week until I had the verdict. I got the sense that she did not appreciate my calling her directly.

Speaking of verdicts, it was in the news that Martha Stewart had decided not to appeal her guilty verdict, but to go to jail as soon as possible so that she might serve her time, get it past her and move on with her life. I could relate to what she was saying and how she felt. I wanted to serve my time and get on with my life too, but for patients with breast cancer the sentence is never over.

So I went back to waiting. For the first time in weeks, I put on my wedding band and rings. I had taken them off because you cannot wear any metal during an MRI, and it seemed that I was down there so often there was no point in wearing them. Having removed the symbols of being in a marriage seemed to reinforce my sense of aloneness. Because, no matter how supportive Bobby was, he could not, like the rings, come into the MRI with me or lie beside me on that table. No matter how much support he could offer, in the end I felt alone with my disease.

Jenna arrived home with the expected university laundry and friends in tow. The house was rocking and rolling with all three kids around. The girls were back in their rooms but the house seemed to have a revolving door with their friends coming and going. It felt familiar and comfortable but at the same time frightening.

Dinner was fun, with Jenna talking a mile a minute (as usual), catching us up on university gossip, her classes and her new apartment. It was more than a little humorous to hear her complain about roommates who didn't wash their dishes or pick up after themselves: her room at home always looks like a hurricane has struck. You don't see it that way when it is yours. She reminded me of myself at her age.

Morning, and the kids were getting ready for synagogue. I would not be going. I was in my feeling-sorry-for-Marla mode. The girls were screaming over wearing each other's clothes. I was screaming at them too and my husband told me I was being a witch. I knew he was right. I wished someone would pass me my broom to fly away. When they got home, Matt asked me why I couldn't come to lunch. I was resting with my arm over my head and he looked shocked as he asked if that was a cut under my arm. He looked so scared. I told him it was but that I was fine, I would be going to lunch. Get up, Marla. Stop being such a witch.

On Friday afternoon Amanda headed out with her fellow newly named prefects from her all-girls school to Outward

Bound—a good break for her. Jenna and I and a close friend in whom she had confided headed out to shop—a distraction at best. I immersed myself in Jenna's quest for the ultimate jeans and did find myself distracted. At 4:30 we had bumped into Renee by happenstance when my phone rang. It was David, my surgeon. He asked me if I was driving and, if so, to pull over. *Oh great. Pull over.* My heart dropped to my feet and I asked him if I should be worried—obviously only a rhetorical question. "A little," he said, and I could feel my heart rate climb and my head feel light.

He told me what I already knew in my gut: there was no longer any doubt about micro-invasion; it had been confirmed. Not all of the breast tissue had been sectioned—the examinations were still in progress—but he did have some preliminary information. He knew nothing about the size of the tumour, if the margins were clear or the extent of the invasion. He did not know if the whole tumour was grade 3 or if there were "better," lower-grade tumours along the way. But he was clearly more concerned now about the nodes and no longer trusted the frozen sections taken from the OR: he wanted special stains done to be sure that the nodes were in fact clear. We also didn't know a thing about the left breast yet; it was not his immediate concern, as the biopsy had not shown cancer on that side. He reminded me that if only a small part in the right breast proved to be invasive, he would not recommend chemotherapy. I was not prepared to play the what-if game. I needed to know and I would not know until the pathology was complete. I was not surprised, but worried that there would be more devastating news waiting for me in the next few days.

That call was clearly hard for David to make. Months later we would sit down and talk about this and I would hear exactly how difficult it was for him. Much like me, Dr. McCready prefers to deliver news in person, especially bad news. We both know the phone is not a good way to give bad news. But he also knew that I had been waiting close to 10 days for some kind of indication. He would tell me that when the pathology became available late on a Friday he knew there was no way to reach me and get me downtown in person. There were only two options at that point: let me agonize over the weekend with no news, or make the call. Knowing me personally, he decided that telling me by phone was the lesser of two evils. Still, I appreciated that it was difficult for him. Giving bad news is hard. Giving it to someone you know is even harder.

I told David to please go ahead and book me with a medical oncologist and radiation oncologist so I could have everything lined up. I knew I would want an opinion from an oncologist. We discussed where I should go and decided that I was most comfortable at Princess Margaret Hospital. After the call, I was anxious and upset. Jenna found me sitting outside in the car; she knew the phone call had been bad news. I had a frank conversation with her in front of her girlfriend as we headed over to my girlfriend Anne's. My rash was driving me nuts. I said that I was dying of itch and somehow she thought I had said I was a dying bitch. We laughed cautiously at our macabre humour.

That evening I sat with Bobby and went over everything. I was anxious and finding it hard to stay in the moment and be optimistic. I remembered when I was having trouble getting pregnant—all I could see were pregnant women. Now, similarly, all I could see were grandmothers and the elderly, and I envied their age and survival. Without the complete pathology report, I could not help feeling that I was drowning. I didn't have a plan. I didn't have a life. I felt out of control.

The weekend passed as best it could. Friends came over to visit and we ate the goodies I had baked for the holidays. Bobby remarked that he loved one cake in particular, then asked if I could make more and start freezing them now, just in case I was not around to bake them in the future. I get his sense of humour, so I told him I would get right on it.

Later that night Jen came downstairs to tell us that Matt had asked her if I was fighting breast cancer. Not knowing what to say, she had said nothing to him. We waited a day, then tried to open the door to a discussion but he denied having any questions or concerns. I knew that once I had a treatment plan we would have to talk to him.

And at long last I made that dreadful call to my parents. I felt I could no longer withhold the information from them. My parents had already endured the death of a grandchild. My mother would often say that this was not the way things were supposed to happen—grandparents should not outlive their grandchildren. I knew my parents would again be thinking about outliving a younger generation—this time, their own daughter. My father was very upset and kept the conversation short. My mother could not get on the phone. I knew she must have been shocked and overwhelmed by her own fear and anxiety. I am my mother's daughter. I knew this would envelop and destroy them—and yet I would feel responsible for keeping them well, just as I always had. I did not want this responsibility, at least not now, as I was trying to keep my own head above water. I was angry and disappointed, as much for them as for me, that they could not offer any physical support to either me or my kids. But what could I expect? They live in another province, and truly there was not much they could do for me. And I realized that by having moved away all those years ago, I was not there to support them either.

It was impossible for them, being so far away and letting their imaginations play out their worst fears. Four days would go by before my father could pick up the phone, and I knew he did so only because I had been ranting to my sister. I would not hear from my mother for several more days. I knew it wasn't because they didn't love me. They didn't know what to say. After that initial conversation, I found myself choking back tears of fear and anxiety for the first time in a few days.

As the weekend came to an end I realized that I had developed cellulitis, a skin infection, under my arm. I could think only of flesh-eating disease—a ridiculous thought, but I was of the mind that only bad news was defining my course. I started an antibiotic, resenting that I was acting as my own doctor but finding it so much easier, at this moment, to go ahead with what I knew I would ultimately be told. And I realized how hard this weekend had been for Jenna. She was getting ready to go back to university, and because I was afraid of crying yet again in front of her, I sent her an e-mail. I told her that I would be fine. Later, she sent a reply:

> Mama, you are the strongest person I know and there is no doubt in my mind that you will fight this. I love you and I know that you will get through this and I am right by your side for whatever you need. I love you so much. You say screw it and so do I. You are better than cancer and you will show it who's boss!!!! If there is anything that I have learnt from you, it is definitely that no one messes with you . . . not even breast cancer. I love you.

I told myself to clean up my attitude. *I have a war to win. Not everyone dies from this damn disease. Get it in check.*

On Monday I returned to the office; it was sheer relief to have a reason to get up and get dressed, to have a destination and purpose. I could not underestimate the value of work for me: slipping into that professional role is the best coping mechanism there is. While I could not overtly deny to myself what was happening, immersing my brain into what I do allowed me to deny that part of my reality for a few hours. There were endless reports to go through, letters, phone calls to return and patients to re-book. I was so out of control, so very much *not* in charge of what was happening in my body, that it was great to be in charge of my work life.

My office staff and I tried to figure out how we should schedule the coming weeks but we were all feeling somewhat helpless, not knowing what would happen to me in the near future. Knowing that there was invasion and fearing that it was extensive, I was imagining chemotherapy and time away. I was beginning to realize that I might not be able to return to *Balance* if I was in the midst of chemo. But there was nothing to say yet. I had no firm news. I was not ready to do anything without a plan. The day went by—no word from my surgeon.

SIX

And the Oscar goes to ...

Day 13, and I still had no formal results from pathology. I was at the end of my patience. I had decided that if there were no results by Wednesday I would call pathology and nudge gently, no matter how unwelcome I might be. It was hard to find that space between being the patient and a doctor.

Finally, I gave in. I called pathology and simply asked when the results would be ready. The secretary told me they had just been posted. I resisted the temptation to have them faxed over and instead called David McCready. Within the hour he called to say that he was in the OR but had looked at the computer posting of my results. It was clear he had not yet been able to read it in its entirety, since he was between cases, but he could tell me that the area of invasion looked good. He also let me know that he'd been unsuccessful in finding me an oncologist at PMH and suggested I move over to Sunnybrook Hospital. I agreed, since Sunnybrook is much closer to my home. I had also met Dr. Maureen Trudeau, who works as an oncologist at Sunnybrook, and while I did not know her well I somehow felt that she and I would be able to connect on various levels. I asked David's secretary to send over the report.

A short time afterwards I tracked down my radiologist, Dr. Bukhanov, who sounded much less optimistic than Dr. McCready had. She pointed out that the left breast, the one without the tumour, was atypical, with abnormal-looking cell precursors and a risk of future malignancy. In fact, later it would be identified as lobular carcinoma in situ, which was not cancer now but a marker for future cancer risk. Knowing how dense my breast tissue was, I was immediately concerned that an early tumour was lurking there without the mammogram or MRI picking it up. Karina agreed this was not an unreasonable thought and I sensed her concern. She also pointed out that on the side with the malignancy there was a very small anterior margin. What that meant was that the ductal carcinoma in situ—the non-invasive part and the lesser of the two cancerous evils—was only 1 millimetre from the anterior skin margin, that margin of skin closest to the front of the breast. The only way to make that margin larger was by removing more tissue and skin. (David would tell me later that a 1-millimetre margin for an in situ lesion is more than adequate.) Karina said that in order to have any sense of certainty in the future, I would need mammograms, alternating with MRIs, every six months. I knew what that really meant, and for the first time I could honestly see that a bilateral mastectomy was a viable and likely option. The vulnerability of my left breast—the "healthy" breast—might have gone unnoticed if we had not pushed for the second biopsy, and this realization made me somewhat angry. But what else was new? Dr. Bukhanov also told me that the pathologists had had trouble identifying exactly how many invasive foci there were, which would be critical to my future management. It was the number of invasive foci that would determine the recommendation for chemotherapy. My head was reeling.

Shortly thereafter the geneticist called to tell me that the common Ashkenazi Jewish gene deletions were negative. We would go forward and do the more extensive testing but it was unlikely to be positive. I breathed a sigh of relief for both myself and my children. I would not have to remove my ovaries, and I now knew that while my children faced a higher risk than the average population because their mother had breast cancer, it was not the much higher risk of those who carry the BRCA mutation.

The pathology report was faxed over to me but I ignored it. I finished the day at the office and then, at home, read the 10 pages of the report. The pathologist had been methodical, but based on the slices of tissue and how the slides had been prepared I could see that she could not be accurate.

Imagine, if you will, a chocolate-chip cake. Now imagine slicing that cake. Each piece will vary in the number of chocolate chips you have, but it is only the chocolate chips you are interested in. A narrow piece means you get fewer; you have missed getting the area you wanted. Another way of imagining this is to think of putting a stick through a loaf of bread and then slicing the loaf. In each individual slice it looks as if these are individual pieces of stick. It is hard to know that the pieces all came from the same stick. So too with slicing breast tissue: representative samples of the breast are taken but the entire breast cannot be examined. From representative slices of breast tissue the pathology is read.

The pathology report told me a number of things. It was clear from the special stains that the three nodes sampled were negative. The in situ carcinoma, the "good news" tumour that was localized, was in fact a grade 3 out of 3. That was irrelevant, other than to remind me that a grade 3/3 is the most aggressive and likely to spread. Had it not spread or invaded, radiation would have been all that was immediately necessary and there would have been a risk of local recurrence. But in my case the grade 3/3 had invaded. There was some debate about the overall size of the in situ carcinoma but it was clearly larger than the 1.6 centimetres the mammogram called, and smaller than the 4.5 centimetres or so that the MRI called. There were several invasive foci and the invasive cancer was moderately aggressive, at a grade of 2/3. The pathologist also noted that there were occasional foci of "lymphovascular permeation." It was an odd term from my point of view—"permeation" sounds much kinder than "invasion." It is the invasion into lymphatic systems or vascular blood systems that puts you at risk for disease at distant sites and ultimately for the cancer's spread to bone, brain and liver. And that, of course, is what finally does you in.

The invasive ductal carcinoma was identified in four adjacent slides but the pathologist stated that it was not possible to determine with accuracy the number of foci of invasion. I could not believe what I was reading. Although I knew it was common to not always be clear, we needed the best and most accurate estimate—my life would depend on it. According to the report, some areas appeared separate but some were presumed to be continuous, in a plane. That plane might not have been visible from the sections we had. Not every plane of breast cancer could be sectioned. However, in the plane that had been sectioned and seen, the dimensions varied from 0.7 millimetres to 3.4 millimetres. The total estimate of invasion was not given and this was the data I needed. If these areas were unrelated areas of invasion, merely separate parts that had invaded on their own at different times, the news would be better. But if in fact these areas of invasion were all part of the same stick, if you will . . . well, then it was not looking good.

The receptors of the tumour were noted. Receptors essentially tell you how the tumour is fuelled or fed. I was indeed estrogen- and progesterone-positive between 30% and 60% of the time. That meant that I would have to be put into menopause and managed, over the long term, with an anti-estrogen drug called tamoxifen and eventually with a newer class of medications called aromatase inhibitors, which stop conversion of peripheral hormones in the bloodstream to estrogen. The good news in this regard is that I am Her-s/neu protein overexpression-negative, and that is a more favorable indicator of my future health. It sounds complicated, for sure, but what the medical community has learned as time has gone on is that each breast cancer is its own disease. We now can type receptors such as estrogen and progesterone to help guide treatment options, and as well we can now measure a certain kind of protein. These advances have helped shape treatment regimens. Because I am Her-s/neu protein–negative I would not be a candidate for a newer drug called Herceptin.

The specimen of the left breast, my healthy breast, was in fact not so healthy. The pathology showed markers for risk of future malignancy. There was a complete spectrum of atypia, from ductal atypia to lobular atypia. Bear in mind that the breast is made of ducts and lobules, and though "atypia" meant they were not normal, it also means they were not malignant—at least not yet. None of the tissue was normal. This told me what I already knew: I was at risk for breast cancer. I was already there.

That night I called Dr. Susan Love, whom I had met previously and visited in California, where she lives and works. She is a wonderful, forthright oncologist, a leader in her field. She got back to me immediately and spent a great deal of time on the phone with me. She pointed out that if there were few areas of invasion, then either radiation or a mastectomy were options, with tamoxifen. If there were more areas of invasion, the situation would change. She was blunt in pointing out what I already knew, that chemotherapy was not without risks and side effects, and she could not recommend it unless I really needed it. There were long-term risks of cardiac toxicity and permanent heart damage, future risk of leukemia and also "chemo brain"—a term that has been applied to those who have been treated with chemotherapy and end up with a change in their memory and sometimes cognitive, or thinking, function. When my friends and I were all pregnant, we used to joke about pregnancy brain—the forgetting of things, the not being clear. Chemo brain was worrisome. Then, of course, there was simply getting through chemotherapy, which itself can kill you. We also talked about bilateral mastectomy as an option. Her best advice was to get a second read on the pathology, recognizing that the report was excellent in its preparation but perhaps a second opinion would help us be more accurate. She asked who I was seeing in Canada and was delighted to hear that I would be seeing Dr. Maureen Trudeau at Sunnybrook Hospital, an oncologist who happens to have trained under Dr. Love at the Dana-Farber Cancer Institute in Boston, Massachusetts.

I called Dr. Trudeau at Sunnybrook the next day; she had already heard from David McCready, my surgeon, for which I was so grateful. She had a copy of the pathology report and immediately saw the dilemma. She told me she wanted the tissue for another read. The pathology had been done at Princess Margaret and was exemplary in the expertise of how it was done and who read it, but it wouldn't hurt to get another opinion.

I arranged to pick up the slides and blocks by hand, as I could not trust my life to a courier service. Dr. Trudeau told me to take it easy and arranged to see me after the weekend, Monday morning at 11. She mentioned that many of her patients watched my show and perhaps it would be best to come on an "off" day, Monday, rather than Tuesday or Wednesday, which were the days of the week when she saw her breast cancer patients. I was grateful for her empathy.

I spent the weekend poring over the pathology, wondering what would have happened had I done my mammogram at the 12-month mark rather than the 18-month mark. Perhaps there would be no invasion. At this suggestion, my husband pointed out that perhaps they would not have seen anything then, and at 24 months it might have progressed to positive lymph nodes. I agreed not to persevere in that line of thinking . . . it was not so easy to let go, but I did.

A study came out that weekend from the National Cancer Institute in the U.S., which told a story that was essentially like mine. This is the summary, from a medical site that reviews the studies:

Breast density, rapid tumour growth contribute to mammogram failure in women in their forties

Lower sensitivity of mammography in women aged 40 to 49 years compared with older women can be largely explained

by greater breast density and rapid tumour growth in the younger women, according to a new study in the October 6 issue of the Journal of the National Cancer Institute.

Because mammography is imperfect for women in their 40s, there has been controversy over whether and how often these women should be screened. Mammographic sensitivity—that is, the percentage of cancers detected by a mammogram—is lower in this group of women than in older women. Several factors have been suggested as contributing to the lower mammographic sensitivity, including higher breast density, faster tumour growth rate, and differences in the distribution of breast cancer risk factors.

To analyze the relative contributions of these factors to differences in mammographic sensitivity between younger and older women, Diana S. M. Buist, Ph.D., of Group Health Cooperative in Seattle, and colleagues studied 576 women (73 aged 40 to 49 years and 503 aged 50 years and older) who were diagnosed with invasive breast cancer between 1988 and 1993. They looked at associations between potential explanatory factors and the odds of having an interval cancer (cancer diagnosed within 12 or 24 months after a negative screening mammogram and before a subsequent mammogram).

Interval cancers occurred in 27.7% of the younger women and 13.9% of the older women within 12 months of a screening mammogram and in 52.1% of younger women and 24.7% of older women within 24 months. Greater breast density—which has been shown to reduce mammographic quality—explained 67.6% of the decreased mammographic sensitivity in younger women at 12 months. Rapid tumour growth explained 30.6% and greater breast density explained 37.6% of the decreased sensitivity in younger women at 24 months. The authors suggest that screening younger women at yearly intervals may reduce the adverse impact on mammographic sensitivity of rapid tumour growth that occurs in young women.

"There are 21.7 million women in the United States aged 40–49 years, approximately 50% of whom have dense breasts," the authors write. "It may be that digital mammography, computer-aided detection, magnetic resonance imaging, and/or ultrasound can improve cancer detection in women with dense breast tissue."

Of course, that was me: mid-40s, breasts that were dense, rapid tumour growth. Nice to know I fit in with the overall population; I was not unique. But again it fuelled my anger at the lack of resources and availability of MRI in Canada and the fact that MRI had not been offered to me as another screening tool before I developed invasive breast cancer.

I went with Bobby to see Dr. Trudeau on Monday. While waiting at the sign-in desk with my husband, with my back to the seating area, several women began to loudly speculate if I was *that* doctor, the one with the TV show *Balance*. Among themselves they discussed which one would come and ask for an autograph. My husband was uncomfortable for me, but I was fine; I told him it was a reflection of the show's popularity, which was great. Then, a few seconds later, one very audibly asked, "Do you think she has cancer?" Bobby was horrified, the secretary was horrified and I was stunned at the comment. My outrage had nothing to do with who I was on any level, but rather with this woman's lack of respect for another person's privacy. I wanted to turn around and yell, "Yes, I do have cancer, but guess what? I am not deaf." The secretary moved us along into a room and apologized. I assured her it was fine. It was becoming clear that I would not be able to do this anonymously. It was impossible.

Dr. Trudeau came in, pathology report in hand, and I delivered to her my precious cargo: my breasts and slides in a box. Based on her reading of the pathology report from Princess Margaret, she had considered both a best-case scenario of minimal invasion and a worst-case scenario of aggressive invasion. She told me that when she read the report and tried to put it together with the mammograms and MRI reports she felt I was neither best case nor worst case, but somewhere in between. Having said that, she felt I was closer to the worst-case scenario and chemotherapy was required.

The worst-case scenario looks like this: healthy baseline patient, 48 years old, ER status (the receptors) positive, tumour size from 2.1 to 3.0 centimetres, no positive nodes. The prognosis for that untreated is (sitting down?) 21% mortality—death—in 10 years. That is one in five and I was blown away. Essentially that means, with no additional therapy, 77.1 women out of 100 will be alive in 10 years, 20.8 will die of cancer and 2.1 will die of other causes. With hormonal therapy such as tamoxifen and aromatase inhibitors, 5.4 more will be alive. With chemotherapy, 6.9 more will be alive, and with combined therapy, 10.6 more will be alive—roughly a 54% improvement in mortality. I hate numbers, as I always tell my patients, but what this told me was that with combined aggressive therapy 87.7 out of 100 women will be alive. Not perfect at all.

When we look at the best-case scenario, the numbers are fantastic: 93.7 out of 100 are alive with a tumour that is between

0.1 and 1.0 centimetre. Watching me, Dr. Trudeau said that I fell somewhere in between these two scenarios. It was clear that I would be having chemotherapy.

We reviewed what she suggested and she thought it was reasonable—necessary, in fact—to be aggressive. She also thought I was healthy enough to have a regimen called "dose-dense," which means higher doses in a shorter interval. It meant I would need daily injections of a medication called Neupogen to support my white blood cell count, which was guaranteed to plummet. Administered every two weeks, the first four treatments would be a combination of Adriamycin (its generic name is doxorubicin, but it's commonly known as "the red devil") and Cytoxan (sometimes known as Procytox and generically called cyclophosphamide). The next four treatments, over the following eight weeks (barring any delays), would be Taxol (generically called paclitaxel), and I knew that would not be a picnic.

We made the arrangements. I had to do *Canada AM* in the morning, then fly to Moncton and Halifax for two days to give talks. I wondered how I would do this. I called my executive producer from *Balance*, Jordan Schwartz, and told him it was urgent we meet. We arranged to meet the next day following *Canada AM*. I had never asked for an urgent meeting, and I am sure he thought I was quitting and moving to New York.

I called my office and let them know that I would be under-going chemo, and that arrangements would have to be made for my patients during the weeks I would be away. (Because my immune system would be compromised by the chemother-apy, I could not be around patients who might have infectious diseases. My office would have been like a landmine to me as I lost my white counts.) I was so fortunate to have a part-time associate, an excellent physician, who could and did take over the practice. My last day was one week away and chemotherapy would start the next day. It didn't seem real. I felt like I was standing on a slippery slope, about to go hurtling down at full speed.

One more appointment: we had to see Dr. McCready for my post-op check. We discussed the pathology report briefly, but he was leaving its interpretation to Maureen, my oncologist. He felt the Taxol was aggressive, but understood her point of view. We also talked about the idea of a bilateral mastectomy. He understood my lack of confidence in future mammograms and MRIs, and my concern about the very real risk of local recurrence for both breasts. A bilateral mastectomy might be a reasonable option, he agreed, but he encouraged me to take time to consider. I told him, yes, I would do that.

We headed home and asked Amanda to sit with us while we called Jenna; we told them the news, couching it as best we could. But the hardest was yet to come: we had to tell Matt. We had to tell Bobby's mother. Then I had to call to update my parents, who had been noticeably silent.

That night we sat down with Matt, and Bobby told him about the breast cancer. We asked him if he knew what it meant and he said yes but it was clear he did not. We told him that in a few weeks I would be bald. He looked positively astounded and asked if I would be getting a buzz cut. I told him the medicine they would give me was strong and one of the ways we'd know it was working was that my hair would fall out. He asked if I would be getting a wig and, more important, if he could try it on. He seemed to be handling it well, but my feelings were overwhelming; I could barely hear myself talking to him, and I could not gauge his response. Everybody sounded so far away.

We called my parents and kept it brief. What was there to say, other than I was a fighter and would be fine?

And then I called Beverly Thomson. Bev is the host of *Canada AM* and formerly a news anchor at a competitor station. Bev had gone public with her breast cancer, and now I wanted her advice. She was terrific, giving me endless time on the phone and pointing out that at the time of her diagnosis, she was seen in an Ontario-only market and I was seen nationally. She encouraged me to make a statement and be in charge of the message rather than let the news slip out without my consent and, perhaps, not as I would have wanted. Bev later told me that she hung up the phone that day and asked herself the same question that countless others would ask: how could this happen to Marla, a doctor? And then she reminded herself that breast cancer does not discriminate. It really does not care if you are a doctor, a journalist or TV host, mother, daughter, teacher, lawyer, whatever. It does not discriminate at all.

Being in charge of the message was important to me. It was indeed the way we all felt, as a family. I called Amanda and Matt back in and got Jenna on the phone, and we told them that this would be public. As a physician and a woman, I felt this was an important message and perhaps it could make a difference. I was not ashamed, embarrassed or reclusive. I was going to share this story. It was important to remind women that breast cancer is still out there.

I told Matt that I had called his best friend's mother to tell her, and he seemed surprised and asked me why. It was not a secret, I replied, and his best friend lives at our house half the time and Matt is at theirs the other half; nothing would change, except that I would be home a whole lot and I wanted everyone to feel all right with this. Later he called his friend to tell him I had breast cancer, and urged him to ask his mom what that meant. It is good advice to try to see the world through your children's eyes, and I knew it would be a relief for my daughters to feel that, to some degree, the cloak of secrecy and privacy could now be lifted. I knew that their friends would be supportive, a relief for them and for me as well.

Breast cancer is not just about the patient; it is a disease that affects the entire family. I was just beginning to see that, albeit in a limited way. While I had asked the kids to keep quiet all this time, it was only with me in mind. I was realizing that their feelings had to be acknowledged and supported and that in many ways they felt just as diseased as I did. Everyone was going to be affected. Everyone already was.

Tuesday morning, and time for my meeting with Jordan Schwartz after *Canada AM*. I headed up to the executive office and sat down with Jordan. I could see that he was already worried by my urgency and my demand for a meeting. He could see this was not about ABC but something more serious. I told him and he was crestfallen. I adore this man who has helped to sculpt my career, and I promised him I would be okay. I joked that it was kind of me to do this during our *Balance* hiatus and breast cancer awareness month, and he chided me for being so flippant. More seriously, I offered to step down from *Balance*, but he would not hear of it. We agreed to ask Mike Cosentino, the publicist for CTV, to come in. We told him what was going on and why I thought it best to issue a simple statement. He listened and let me know I didn't have to do this, but agreed that in the end it would be easiest for me. I told him no one would take notice and he told me I was wrong. We worked on a statement until I felt comfortable with it.

I went down to see Robert Hurst, the president of network news, to tell him, and then to *Canada AM*. I asked Seamus O'Reagan, Bev and my producer, Denise Kimmel, to talk with me for a few minutes. Seamus and Denise looked confused but they followed me into Bev's office. Much to my surprise, just as I was about to start speaking, I became tearful. I had been so good at holding it together. I took a deep breath, regained my composure and told them. In the midst of the shock there were hugs and good wishes, but I threatened them that I would continue to be around and would do my best to make them crazy—daily.

With that, I could hardly breathe anymore. I ran home, grateful to fly off to Moncton.

While at the airport I made a few quick calls to friends who did not yet know, but whom I wanted to inform personally. I also called my former long-time producer from *Canada AM*, now a senior producer at *Balance*, Brent Paszt. He and his wife had just had a baby and I was sure he was wondering why I had not come around yet to see the baby. He started the conversation laughing and asking when I was moving to New York; I quickly let him know what was up. He could hardly believe it.

As I waited to board the plane I received a call from CTV's Sandie Rinaldo, who had just heard the news: she was warm and wonderful and supportive. One last call—to my daughter's high school. Amanda was in her final year, a stellar student and a prefect, and I knew how important her marks were to her. I was so concerned about how this would affect her. I wanted her principal and teachers to know what Amanda was facing. The principal of the senior school, having been in Amanda's position when her husband was ill, was supportive.

After the call, I heard the stewardess asking us to turn off all cellphones. I had never been so grateful to hear those words.

That first night in Halifax, just before 11 p.m., my cellphone rang. It was Lloyd Robertson, the anchor for CTV's nightly news broadcast. In that voice so familiar to so many of us, he told me that he had heard about my cancer and wished me the best for a speedy recovery. I was overwhelmed by the kindness of this gesture, overwhelmed that I was lucky enough to know and work with this impressive man.

For the next two days I was ushered around the maritime provinces, giving talks to physicians and other health care professionals on new osteoporosis medications and management. As with my medical practice, I found it so therapeutic to immerse myself in the medical world and forget about what lay ahead. By Thursday I was back home, with three full, busy days to put in at the office, trying to keep it all together. On Tuesday I would do *Canada AM* and head off to chemo. No free time, and that is how I lived my life. Nothing had changed—yet.

When I arrived home Thursday from my speaking engagements, Dr. Trudeau called to tell me that the reread of the pathology put me in the worst-case scenario. I was incredulous, but confident she was offering me the right regimen.

I also had an appointment with Dr. Joan Lipa, a plastic surgeon who specializes in reconstruction. I knew I was getting ahead of myself, but just as I meticulously research stories for the show and for my patients, I needed to research this. I needed to know all my options. Breast cancer, this slippery slope, is a cascade of fast-paced decision-making. I needed accurate information from the experts. If I was to go the reconstruction route, Dr. Lipa and Dr. McCready would do tag-team surgery: he would remove the breasts, and she would reconstruct.

There were two main options. One is called a TRAM, which stands for the transverse rectus abdominis muscle, located in the lower abdomen between the waist and the pubic bone: in this option, the abdominal tissues, skin and body fat are transplanted, with their own blood supply, up through a flap to create a new breast. I didn't have a lot of fat on my abdomen and although removing fat from the gluteal (buttock) area was possible, it would leave large incisions and deformities, and there too I had little fat to use.

The other option was implants, though I understood this was a long, arduous and painful procedure. After the mastectomy was done, if I opted for that route, shaped expanders would be inserted under the pectoral muscles to stretch the muscles and skin. An implant with a magnetic port would be put into each breast area and gradually, over several months, the port would be filled to a predetermined size. Eventually that bag and the expanders would be removed and a permanent implant inserted. The areola, the dark circle around the nipple, could be transplanted from other skin or tattooed on, and nipples could be fashioned from skin from the ear, labia minora or underarm.

Like Dr. Trudeau, Dr. Lipa asked if my identity as a woman was tied up in my breasts. Both asked this question not with sarcasm but as an honest question that needed to be considered. My answer was that my identity was tied up in my brain—always had been. But I appreciated the question and for the first time ever would have to give it some honest thought. There was a lot to think about, a lot to digest and understand. Dr. Lipa suggested that I go home and simply consider it all.

Friday afternoon I sent out more than 75 personal e-mails to colleagues, and other e-mails cancelling appearances that were booked over the next six months. I realized that they all deserved an explanation and, being as upfront as I am, I tried to be clear: I told them about my diagnosis. "Medical reasons" would have sounded so vague.

Over the next few days I couldn't keep up with the flurry of e-mails and calls and I realized that this response was just the beginning. Friends are wonderful, they really are, and anyone with a chronic disease will quickly get a clear view of the landscape and who the true friends are. So many others who have walked this walk would remind me to surround myself with only positive energy and cut the debris away. Good advice.

People sent e-mails and tried to be supportive, but . . . While no words are ever perfect, I can tell you what is not, or at least was not for me. Anything that began with how sorry they were or used the adjectives *horrendous, terrible, tragic* (you get it?) made me scream. I would send off rockets to those people, re-educating them that cancer is none of the above. It is not a dreadful disease, a scourge or a plague. It is breast cancer and we have the tools to fight it. If I hadn't been so angry, I would have paused and agreed that I too thought this was a dreadful disease. But hearing it from others made it sound hopeless, and my death inevitable.

Bobby and Matt and I escaped to a friend's cottage over the weekend. Amanda had gone to London to see her sister, which relieved me. I hid up north, grateful that no one knew where I was and the cellphone wouldn't work.

At the same time, I heard from the Gemini Awards that I had been nominated in the Viewer's Choice category as most popular host. The public has to cast votes online, although it was totally unclear to me how this contest was publicized. As they say in media, though, there is no bad publicity.

On Monday my good friend and office manager Barb was taking me for a wig fitting. As I left the office, the staff started to cry. I hugged them, told them it would be okay and, my emotions barely intact, ran downstairs.

We met at my house and she insisted we go for lunch. While at lunch I got a call from Amanda's school, telling me she had lice. The poor kid. She was pretty horrified and angry that she had gotten lice on the school trip. She was miserable, and then the school nurse told me we all had to treat our heads. I told her I would get Matt a bean shave—as he had suggested I get—but that I would be bald in a couple of weeks so it hardly mattered. She told me this was serious—perhaps she thought I was saying the lice would eat up my hair. I told her no, but I was starting chemo the next day and would be bald in 14 days. This poor woman, who as it turned out loves *Balance,* just about fell off her chair. I would have to use something less like a sledgehammer in the future. I hung up and laughed so hard I cried. The first positive thing about being bald: I would not have to treat myself for lice!

We went to the wig store, where we were greeted with many choices. I opted for the human hair variety and found a match for my colour. I told the wigmaker, Judy, that I simply wanted to look like me. The wig was tight and uncomfortable but the wigmaker pointed out that I had a ton of hair and when it was all gone the wig would be roomy. She told me that while I still had my own hair and before it began to fall out I should go and have bangs cut. She explained that a wig without a little hair in front looks like a wig, and for that reason the wig would have bangs. She thought it would be a good idea that people get used to me with bangs and my own hair so that the transition would not seem so obvious. Taking her advice I did just that.

Tuesday morning arrived. I went in to CTV, did my report on *Canada AM* and taped the weekend pieces for Newsnet. I snuck out without saying goodbye: I planned on being back the following week. As I left, the statement was released over the wires.

October 5, 2004

The following statement was released today by Dr. Marla Shapiro, medical correspondent for CTV News and Host of CTV's *Balance . . . television for living well.*

"October is Breast Cancer Awareness month in Canada, and I too, like so many other women, will be starting my own personal battle against breast cancer. In fact, today is my first treatment. I have the wonderful support of my family, friends and my colleagues both at my practice and at CTV. Though I plan to continue practicing medicine, I will indeed take a short leave of absence from my medical office. I do look forward to continuing to report for Canada AM, CTV News and CTV Newsnet from time to time. My show *Balance . . . television for living well* will continue to debut new programs each day and we look forward to the continued support of our viewers!"

Sincerely,
Dr. Marla Shapiro
Host of *Balance . . . television for living well*
Medical Consultant CTV

I had the CTV driver take me over to North York General for the last of the genetic profiling and then headed home to do something I had never done on a weekday: I changed into jeans, got in the car and picked up Matt for lunch. He was amazed to see me, and said he was going to like this part of the breast cancer, having me home. Over lunch he asked if I would wear the wig at home. I asked him why and said that I probably wouldn't. He waited and then asked, without looking at me, what I would do when his friends came over. My heart was breaking as I told him I would do whatever he wanted. "Maybe a baseball cap," he said. So he had been thinking about it, and was worried.

Truth be known—I was too.

PART TWO

INSIDE, LOOKING OUT

SEVEN

Chemotherapy is not for wusses

I headed to Sunnybrook Hospital, alone. It was how I wanted it, to be alone. Bobby had a business engagement in the States and I had forced him to go. I told him I knew what would happen—which I did—and there would be ample opportunity for other sessions, worse sessions. My sister promised to come to Toronto, and with that he agreed to go. But the morning of the first chemo, my sister, who has a terrible time flying, just couldn't get on the plane. I knew this was worse for her than for me—she felt that she'd let me down. But I also know she loves me and I truly understood that she just couldn't do it. Amanda was home from school, of course, grounded with lice, so she drove me over. I kissed her and told her I would call when it was over.

I arrived at the hospital with my patient admittance forms filled out. My drug regimen was called "AC," short for the names of the two drugs (Adriamycin and Cytoxan) that were about to become a very large part of my life. One question on the forms asked about any concerns I might have. Most people write about nausea and baldness. I wrote, of course, about pharmaceutical error in dispensing medications and Adriamycin cardio-toxicity. The nurse read this and realized she had her hands full with me.

The nurses were mad that I was alone, mad that I hadn't eaten, and mad that I hadn't drunk enough water—but admitted I looked damn good in my television makeup.

I headed over to chemo and, after five painful needle pokes to start a vein, was told this was going to be tough to do every two weeks. I agreed to have a surgical procedure to insert a line called a portacath under my chest wall, into the subclavian vein. This would leave a semi-permanent port for the nurses to access for chemo. I knew I had crappy veins.

They gave me my anti-nausea pill first. It's called ondansetron, and at $25 per pill I began to see that having cancer is expensive. They also gave me 12 mg of a steroid called dexamethasone to help strengthen the effect of the anti-nausea pill. Common side effects of ondansetron are headache and constipation, so I got the fibre talk, a talk I constantly have with my own patients. I was told that I might also experience dry mouth, dizziness, fatigue, shortness of breath—on and on went the list. The dexamethasone would increase my appetite, encourage fluid retention and make my already dreadful insomnia even worse. These medications would continue for the next three days following chemotherapy. I also got the talk about mouth ulcers and mouth care, how to use baking soda rinses five times per day. This would be a full-time career.

The usual questions were asked: was I pregnant or breastfeeding? No, in fact I was about to be shoved into menopause. The nurses warned me to use adequate birth control (yup, that was a major concern of mine right then. . . . not), to avoid people with chicken pox or shingles and not to go to the dentist. They also warned me about pedicures and manicures with respect to the infection risk if I got cut—okay, practical—and again warned me against taking aspirin or anti-inflammatory medications. They warned me about signs of infection and I appreciated their treating me like a real patient. Fever, chills, cough. Oral ulcerations, nausea and vomiting. And, of course, the inevitable plummet my white cells would take, which is why I would be out of my medical office. Less commonly, there could be side effects of bruising, diarrhea, darkening of skin, hair and nails and, yes—for sure—my urine would be red over the next two days. Urination could be painful and I should drink more water. I promised I would.

From there they infused the Adriamycin—the A in the AC regimen—in a "push," meaning the nurse slowly pushed the drug in over about a 10-minute span.

The push went well and then they started a 45-minute drip of the next drug, Cytoxan—the C in the AC regimen. It carries the same warnings as Adriamycin, the same side effects, except instead of red discoloration in skin and nails, this drug could turn me yellow. Then, of course, there could also be hives and itching, which for an allergic person like me is more worrisome than anything.

What they didn't tell me, but what I have been told by my friend and receptionist Barb, is that the chemo drugs, as they're being administered, give you a feeling of facial fullness and sinus pain. Sure enough, within five minutes it was unbelievable: my head felt like it was going to be blown off. They offered to slow down the drip and told me this sensation would be gone within two hours of stopping the drip. "Carry on," I told them. I wanted it to be done. While I was sitting through the drip, again they reminded me about hair loss . . . in just 14 days. How could I believe that?

As it approached the time to go home, the pharmacist came in with my meds and a cooler with filgrastim, often known as Neupogen. This is the medication that I would have to inject subcutaneously (under the skin) at home. The drug is technically G-CSF, which stands for granulocyte colony-stimulating factor; it helps the white blood cells (the infection-fighting cells, called granulocytes or neutrophils) to rebuild. With dose-dense chemotherapy, such as I was having, the body's white cell counts are sure to drop, a condition known in medicine as neutropenia. (Any medical term that has *-penia* at the end means low.) The Neupogen is meant to help support the white counts and I was to take it every day for a week, beginning on day three after a cycle of chemotherapy. It has to be refrigerated, and to tell you it is expensive . . . well, how does $18,000 (plus or minus) for the duration grab you? We were not sure if private insurance would cover the cost of the drug and we did not qualify for provincial assistance to pay for it.

The pharmacist was meticulous in her advice: do not shake the vial; the liquid should be clear and colourless, without particles floating around, and of course side effects—joint pains, muscle spasms, rash, itching, redness at the injection site and wheezing, as well as a rapid, irregular heartbeat—could all be expected. The pharmacist reminded me about varying the site of injection each time.

As I was almost done, my girlfriend Susan popped in, looking a little trepidatious. I had been clear about unannounced visits. But, truth be known, it was good to see a familiar face.

We went home, and I still felt like me. Wendy, my sister-in-law, dropped over and I read her the riot act. I needed to feel that my home was a safe haven, and if people felt they could just come over unannounced, it was too intrusive. She felt awful, and though I knew she was well-meaning, I had to make the message clear. I simply wanted a phone call. I didn't, at that moment, care that my friends had needs and needed to help me: I wanted to be alone, and I could do this alone. Eventually, I would learn that I didn't have to do it that way, nor should I have. And frankly, as I would come to learn, it is a rather selfish attitude. Still, at the time, I needed to set clear boundaries around my private space, my home.

On the first day after chemo I felt pretty much like my usual self, except that my mouth was dry. Well, that and the fact that every television station across the country, and many newspapers, had picked up my story. That struck me as bizarre, because I do not see myself as a personality or a celebrity, never have. I see myself as a physician who has a lot of fun teaching, only I teach to a broader audience and it is a privilege I do not underestimate.

Again and again the doorbell rang as flowers were delivered—endlessly, it seemed. I put the message out that while I appreciated all the gestures, I would prefer people to make a donation instead. In any case, for women about to become nauseated by chemo, the scent of flowers can tip them over the edge.

The phone was crazy, prompting me to get call display, and the e-mails were coming in by the hundreds. I was overwhelmed. Some of the e-mails were great, others so full of sympathy I wanted to scream, even though I knew the sentiment was coming from the right place. As I read the e-mails and notes my back would go up. Cards that said get well soon would have me firing off a note that I was not sick. At least, I did not feel ill. I had a disease called cancer, but I didn't think of myself as sick. Semantics, I suppose, but I hated to have people thinking of me as ill. A colleague called to offer words of support, and then asked me "how far gone" I was, if my lymph nodes were positive. I marvelled at the stupidity and brashness of some questions that were asked of me. Yes, I had gone public, but what made people think they could ask such personal, invasive or just plain insensitive questions?

But some notes, particularly from my patients, made me sit in wonderment at who they were talking about. Their notes reminded me of things I had done for them and expressed gratitude for events gone by. Letters that told me cancer was messing with the wrong kind of girl made me smile. A note written in grade-one scrawl (complete with a backwards "s") from a little one promising not to get sick until I got better so I could take care of her, made me cry. A note from a patient I had not seen in decades reminded me that when I told her, many years ago, that she had breast cancer, she called me a liar. When I told her she was going to be fine, she called me a liar again, and I told her that, no, she was the liar and all would be well. She wrote to tell me I had been right and that these many years later she was indeed fine—I would be fine too, she assured me. Such letters made me so grateful for the life I led, had—have—and I began to realize that what I was rebelling against was the feeling that cancer had ripped this life away from me. Over and over again I was reminded that the strength I had for my patients was the strength I now had to use for myself.

And as I reacted over and over again to the cards, letters and e-mails that kept arriving in those first days and weeks, I began to realize that there is no "right thing" to say; no words, no matter how much they irritated or angered me, were wrong. The notes and thoughts were all coming from the right place, a place of support. What was worse were the people who could not say anything to me, or looked away. Two close friends had not been in touch since hearing the news. This angered me, until I could take a step back and realize how hard this was for them. I e-mailed them, gently chiding them and reminding them that I was the same person now as before I had cancer, and that I needed their support. I invited them back into my life. Nothing substitutes for clear communication.

One thing became clear to me: I had to let my anger go. I began to realize that my anger was at the cancer, not at those who were sending words or gestures of support. I began to realize that maybe expressions of sympathy made me fearful that I would not beat this. My fears, which were usually below the surface, were nonetheless real and well-informed: as a doctor, I knew too much, had read too much, seen too much, had seen it for too long. Where I could reassure my patients, there was no reassurance for me. Perhaps not surprisingly, I had spent a lot of energy making everyone else feel comfortable, reassuring everyone else that I was fine—I could not let go of my role as a physician.

In terms of my physical reactions to chemo, I wasn't sure now what to expect. I had been warned that in the first 24 hours after chemo I would pee red; the "red devil," Adriamycin, would be concentrated in my bladder. The dexamethasone would give me insomnia. This was true on both counts. I over-hydrated myself, and watched my urine go from red to clear. Sleep was impossible, as the dexamethasone made me feel like I had drunk 12 cups of coffee. Try as I might, I could not sleep.

For the next two days, I still felt fairly normal, managing to get out, grocery shop and carry on sort of normally. My girlfriends hovered as I tried to figure out what to do with my time.

More important, I was trying to discover who Marla was, shorn of her title, her office and the structure that had defined her days for so many years. Would I even like this woman?

I was about to find out.

EIGHT

Dr. Marla, meet Marla

I was supposed to be in Washington at the North American Menopause meetings. This same week, Amanda was being installed as a prefect in the middle division at her school. She had strived for this goal for many years and it was exciting for all of us that she had been elected by her peers and teachers. With my commitment to the conference in Washington, I was going to miss the installation. No surprise: I travelled a fair amount and was always working. In fact, in June, when Amanda was told of the installation, the call came as I was literally heading out to the airport. If there was one nice thing cancer had done for me, it was to have me home for this special day.

The event was being held on Friday of the Canadian Thanksgiving weekend—three days after "chemo one." I was still wondering why my oncologist would not let me go to Washington. I felt fine—sort of. I had been following my doctor's orders to take my ondansetron and dexamethasone twice daily, and as I went to bed on Thursday night I was looking forward to Friday and Amanda's installation. But about two hours after I went to sleep, I was woken by an overwhelming feeling of sickness. Like so many of my patients who search for but fail to find words to describe an elusive symptom, so I struggle to find the words to describe how I felt. My insides felt as if they were bathed in toxic waste, my gut ached, I was nauseated and suddenly overwhelmed by fatigue and weakness. I had been expecting this to happen, but still I was shocked by how suddenly the feelings of sickness came on. I couldn't get out of bed, or even sit up. I couldn't believe how I felt. It was terrifying. Bobby didn't know what to do for me as I tried to figure out if I felt less sick when sitting up or lying down.

Finally, the morning came. Amanda bounded excitedly into our bedroom, dressed in her red kilt and blazer. She took one look at me and stopped dead in her tracks. I was too weak to sit up. She was overwhelmed and worried. I lacked the strength to fill up the syringe with my Neupogen. Being the only one in the house who wasn't terrified at the sight of needles, she would have to help with my daily injection of Neupogen; I didn't have the strength to draw the serum up. She did it for me as Bobby watched. I placed the needle in my thigh, but she had to plunge it in for me.

Tears filled her eyes as she said I should stay home; she realized I couldn't make it after all. I felt even sicker that she had to see this, see me like this, and that I was frightening her. I told her I was okay. She didn't believe me. I didn't believe me. We sent her off to Timothy Eaton Church, where the installation was to take place, and Bobby told her he would be there. He got dressed. I watched—a bystander in my own life.

I couldn't believe how stupid I had been—to choose a conference over this incredible event for Amanda. I had been so incredibly selfish, telling myself that I had no choice when in fact I had made a choice to go to the conference. Yet again I had chosen career over family without really stopping to think about the impact of my decisions. In my own way, without saying it or even realizing it, I had chosen work as the priority when emotionally, first and always, my children are my priority. Clearly my behaviour did not show that. I was overwhelmed with disbelief at what I had done. And here I was, actually home, and I could not go. This was a painful, cruel lesson. I was willing to learn the lesson, but not willing to pay the price. At 8:30 I forced myself out of bed, put myself together and, over Bobby's objections but also with his help, got myself into the car.

The pomp and ceremony of the installation were awesome, and as Amanda walked in with her peers, everyone rose in unison. I couldn't. I struggled to have her see me but she saw only her father, not me, and I could see how upset she was by the way her expression fell. I sat quietly, willing her to find me in the benches filled with people. Her name was called and she received her pin and was announced as the incoming prefect of the middle division. As she turned around to face the audience, I could literally feel a force pushing me up. I stood up and she saw me. Her face lit up and I was overwhelmed and started to cry silent tears. Cancer—it is not only my disease, but the entire family's. Never had that been so clear. I sat proudly, feeling prouder of my daughter in that moment than of any accomplishment of my own. In an instant, I realized how fearful I was that cancer would rob me of future moments like this. I also realized that my children had exactly the same fears. I could not reassure them away. I could not will them away. Much as I wanted to protect them, I could not.

After the ceremony came a brief reception, and then— finally—home, where I could collapse. It was Thanksgiving weekend and Jenna would be home. Try as I might to will myself into wellness for her arrival, I just could not. I was thrilled to see her but now glued to the couch in the family room. I couldn't join them for dinner; they were heading off to have dinner with Bobby's brother and sister-in-law, Alan and Wendy. I couldn't move, much less eat anything.

Saturday found me in the same state, exhausted and unable to move. I tried to shower but had to sit on the shower floor. The day passed in a haze as I drifted in and out of sleep. Later that evening, Jenna's and Amanda's friends descended on the house as they always do and I forced myself to sit up and join in their company. I didn't want any of them to see me ill, or for Jenna to feel that she could not have her friends over on a visit home from university. She was being sensitive to the way I felt, but I wanted her to feel that we still had a welcoming home. I encouraged Jenna's girlfriends in from Montreal to stay with us. Jenna had been too anxious to ask me if they could stay, so I took the initiative and insisted that the door was open, as always. I found myself buoyed by the giggles and laughter, and for a few moments I managed to be as close as I could remember to who I was before this all started.

The next morning, Sunday, I struggled downstairs and tried to prepare for Tuesday's *Canada AM* and Newsnet tapings. But I couldn't read or concentrate and found myself entirely panicky—I just couldn't do it. I sat there with tears running down my face. It was one thing to be on hiatus (I still couldn't bring myself to say medical leave) from the office, but if I couldn't read, what would become of me? I was overwhelmed, frightened, and I didn't know what to do. I had tenaciously hung on to the *Canada AM* appearances despite the full support of the network to do what I could, when I could. But I was having none of that. Denial is a great tool for coping and I was the queen of denial.

Thankfully, Monday found me feeling somewhat better. As the day went on, the feeling of sickness began to lift, almost as suddenly as it had begun. By Monday night, when Jenna had to go back to London, I was stronger, more functional, more me, though a few pounds thinner.

I was still, though, having a terrible time with the side effects of the ondansetron, one of which is constipation. Because it's not often talked about, I had no clue how horrific this would be. Bowel movements were almost impossible and felt like I was passing shards of glass. I would sit and cry and bleed. Bran, milk of magnesia, Senokot, suppositories—nothing helped. For women going through chemotherapy and using ondansetron, it is important to know this. It is a wonderful drug that allows you to handle the nausea, but the side effects can be overwhelming in their own way.

When Jenna got back to university she called me, tearful and in a full state of panic at having had to leave me. Painstakingly, I reviewed the entire weekend with her, reminding her that in fact it wasn't all that bad, that I was okay, was going to be okay and that the first weekend was the worst weekend. By the time I got off the phone she was feeling better but again I was reminded of the impact this was having on everyone. I felt guilty and angry.

Later that night, Matt asked me if cancer was something that just went away or something that I had to fight. He reminded me that a cold just goes away. Would this just go away? I told him no, it was something I had to fight. Shortly thereafter, and even now, I would see him walking around the house boxing imaginary demons when he thought no one saw him. From his nine-year-old perspective, he was fighting along with me.

On Tuesday I was off to *Canada AM,* where I put on a good show. The host, Bev Thomson, started the segment by asking me how I was doing. I reassured her that I was fine and said I felt it was important for women everywhere to see that you could carry on and have a life and a career even while being treated for cancer: it doesn't have to rob you of your ability to be who you are. I told her it was important for my mother in Montreal to know I was okay. For the first time in 11 years of on-air appearances, I actually waved to my mother.

After that I had an appointment for the final wig fitting. I sat in disbelief as they put something like a wet rat on my head. Then again, think about it—when was the last time you had your hair cut dry? I sat there for an hour as the stylist re-created me. The wig was the same colour as my own hair, the same cut as mine, but I sat there grumpy and unhappy. The hairdresser was patient and empathetic, having walked this mile a few times before. She told me how important it was that I had come in now—before I had lost my hair—so that I could be in control of how the wig looked and not be in a frantic state after the fact. So many women refuse to believe that they will lose their hair, she told me, and finally come in miserable and angry, which makes it harder to be happy with the results. Still, here I was with a full head of hair and I was unhappy, even as I marvelled at how perfect the wig was, how normally it moved. I christened it Judy, the name of the hairdresser who so patiently cut my hair and spoke so kindly to me. I looked like me but I sure as hell did not feel like me. We put her on a wig stand, bought a carrying case and I paid for my new friend. I was shocked at how much it cost. A letter from my physician stating that I needed it for medical reasons meant that the tax would be waived, but still it was inordinately expensive. My advice? If you are undergoing chemo and are going to lose your hair, this is one place not to skimp. You will be wearing this wig for quite some time. It is a necessity, not a luxury, so do it right. It is important to feel like you *can* look normal. It then becomes up to you to define what that new normal might be. For me it was constantly evolving.

I had a goal. (Big surprise. I am very goal oriented—Type A-plus, some would say.) The coming weekend was my 25th reunion for McGill's medical school. I was desperate to go. It would also be an excellent opportunity to see my parents while I still had my hair and looked good. My oncologist, Dr. Trudeau, told me that if my counts were acceptable, I could go. It meant a plane ride, and an airplane is not a good place for an immuno-suppressed person to be. Immuno-suppression simply meant that without my white fighter cells, my immune function was suppressed. I was indeed a sitting duck.

Wednesday morning I went for a blood count and was shocked at the results. My white count had plummeted. I had no neutrophils, the fighter cells that are essential to keeping us healthy. My oncologist said to come in for an extra shot of Neupogen. She advised me to travel midday, when the plane was more likely to be empty, and to take carry-on bags to minimize my time at the airport. Gratefully, but somewhat tentatively, I booked the ticket.

I was scheduled to be a keynote speaker at the reunion but had cancelled my appearance when I assumed I could not go. I arrived in Montreal, and as my parents picked me up I realized how great it was to be there. They were relieved to see me and I was so happy to see them.

The next morning I went down to McGill. Entering the lecture room that I had sat in so many years ago overwhelmed me. Finding my classmates some 25 years later, older, some so changed I had to look at their badges to know who they were, made me feel emotional. I sat down with the same group of women in the exact same seats that we had first sat in so anxiously some 29 years ago. Where had the time gone? And what had happened?

The morning went quickly and although I was not on the speakers list I was asked to make some closing remarks. As I walked down to the podium from the upper rows I wasn't sure what I was going to say. I found myself staring up at a sea of faces and I thanked them for letting me speak. I told them that in my other life, closing a show was called being the kicker. The kicker was *not* what you wanted to be, since most people would nod off by the end of the late-night news. Except, I told them, when the news was exceptional and then you wanted to be the kicker because everyone would remember what you had said. I told them that in this case, following a morning of exceptional speakers, it was an honour to be the kicker. And an honour to come back after all this time and be part of this incredibly accomplished group of men and women. But I cautioned them that our academic and professional life was only part of who we were and that as the weekend went on, it was important to take the time to share who we had become as individuals, who our families were, to share pictures of the kids and leave the academics behind. I told them that with my new challenges, I had come to realize how much the four years at McGill had shaped me and defined me, socially and professionally, as well as personally. As I struggled to leave that behind for a period of time, I explained, I was finding it challenging to rediscover me. I now challenged them, for at least a weekend, to join me in that process.

As the two days passed, I found myself growing more emotional than I had been since all of this had started. Part of me was amazed at how many people I did not remember. Had I been so self-obsessed as a young kid entering medical school, crazed with making it, that I had not taken the time to get to know these people? And part of me simply welcomed old friends back into my life, remembering that they had shared a unique time with me, a time that had changed all of us and sculpted us into who we had become as adults. The girl who entered medical school at 18 was not the woman who had emerged at 22. And it certainly was not the woman I thought I knew. I was just as driven as I had been back then. I was grateful to the life that McGill medical school had made possible for me and the opportunities for which it had trained me. A number of us agreed that e-mail would allow us to stay in touch—had it been there when we graduated, in 1979, so many of us would not have let the bonds of friendship fall away.

As I said goodbye and readied myself to fly home, I found myself in tears, along with my old friends. My girlfriend living in California couldn't understand why she was crying, though she assured me it was not because of the breast cancer; she knew I would be all right. She, like I, was overwhelmed with how we felt, where the time had gone and how our lives had changed since we last stood together as a class. Life had changed since we had tossed our hats up in the sky, future bound.

I boarded the plane to return home to my family and my life as I now knew it. I tried to reconcile everything I was feeling, but try as I might I couldn't, and realized that I needed time. Time to figure out how I felt, who I really was.

NINE

The rhythm of my life

Tuesday, time for *Canada AM* and my second round of chemo. It was clear that this two-week cycle would now define my life. The rapid plummet down, the slow climb back up. I was just back to feeling almost normal. I was just back to being able to eat a little bit. Familiar foods tasted foreign, nothing looked good, coffee made me throw up, and the thought of a great glass of Cabernet was enough to make me run, albeit not all that quickly.

Bobby was with me, having been annoyed at my decision to go to the first chemo alone. I had an appointment at Sunnybrook at 10, right after *Canada AM*, to install a portacath. My veins were impossibly small and chemo number one had been so difficult because of the numerous attempts it required to get an intravenous started.

A portacath, as I mentioned in a previous chapter, is a device that allows access to the vascular (blood) system. There are two different types to consider. One is a small catheter or flexible tube that is placed in your arm and has a port with a special lock. It has to be flushed weekly with heparin, a blood

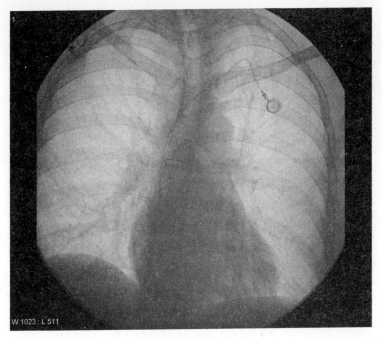

My chest x-ray, with portacath in place

thinner, and has a risk of falling out or becoming infected. With this particular one, although the insertion is easier, it has the disadvantage for the patient of not being allowed to shower. This was not for me.

The second option is a small metal chamber that is topped by a plastic disc. It is placed under the skin and a small tube feeds into a large vein. It is made to withstand between 1,000 and 2,000 needle pricks—not such a pleasant thought. Unlike the first option, it requires two incisions. The procedure begins with an antibiotic and a relaxant being administered, and takes about an hour, under local freezing. I chose this option.

The radiologist who specializes in invasive procedures was introduced to me. Her name was Dr. Robyn Pugash. There had been a Pugash in my medical class and I asked her if they were related. It was her brother. I immediately relaxed and we joked that despite my non-existent white count I had made the reunion but he had not! I told her to e-mail him and tell him. She reassured me that she had done countless procedures like this and it was second nature to her. We looked at the different sizes of portacath and chose, because of my small frame and the weight loss, one of the smaller devices. My particular model was called a P.A.S. Port System. It was made of silicone and titanium and measured 24.5 millimetres by 18.2 millimetres.

From there we went to chemotherapy. My weight had dropped another six pounds and my oncologist reviewed why I was having trouble eating. She asked me to take the dexamethasone a few days longer to stimulate my appetite but I was reluctant. The side effect of insomnia was intolerable, and I was concerned about bone loss and osteoporosis. We agreed that I would continue with the ondansetron and dexamethasone as per the first course, but would add on a proton pump inhibitor medication that is usually used for ulcer treatment. I had been plagued by mouth sores the latter half of the second week and she felt that was reflecting some gastric irritation as well, which might be affecting my appetite. She also offered me a motility agent called domperidone that I would take four times a day. She told me that if I could not maintain my weight my dose would be lowered. Bobby chimed in about my lack of eating and I promised to give it a go. I went off to chemo, sore from the incisions in my chest wall. The freezing was wearing off and I could feel the pain radiate to my neck. But the portacath made it much easier to take the chemo. My potions were mixed and the second round began. My girlfriend Anne joined me as Bobby went home because Matt had called: he had fallen at school and hurt his side and he was now home, upset and crying.

I went home at 6 p.m., round two over. At least this time I knew what to expect.

The immediate side effects were about the same: red urine, headache, loss of appetite and, of course—speedy, speedy. I knew sleep was never going to happen, at least not for the first or second night. I was prepped with lots of reading material. I got home to find countless e-mails telling me Melissa Etheridge had announced that she had breast cancer. Another member of the club. I found it interesting that everyone wanted to tell me this news. One year later, I would be in New York, interviewing her about her new album and the songs "I Run for Life" and "This Is Not Goodbye." Who could have known where this journey would take me?

The new medication made this second round of side effects a little easier. It seemed to push the nausea and side effects along a few days and they were somewhat milder. I could also work, which was something I could not do after the first round.

One item of business, a new one for me, was writing my first column for the *Globe and Mail*. I had been asked previously to become a health columnist, but I'd never had time. I now had time. In my house we joked that after I was diagnosed with cancer, the first call I made was to Bobby and the second was to the *Globe and Mail* to accept their earlier offer. Sylvia Stead, deputy editor of the *Globe and Mail*, put me in touch with my editor, Kathryn Maloney. Kathryn and I agreed that the articles would not be breaking medical news but my point of view on health and lifestyle issues. I wasn't sure that I could write but I agreed to give it a go—another door I was about to walk through.

I sent in the column during the week. It was scheduled for publication the following Tuesday. I was a little nervous—okay, a lot nervous. The first column was about why and how I had decided to try and write for the *Globe and Mail*. It didn't seem possible to introduce myself as a new columnist without explaining why and how I had gotten to that position. But it also meant retelling what was happening to me in another public way. It was also the first time that an editor dissected what I had to say, challenging me to do it better, more concisely. While I found the challenge at times intimidating, it also forced me to focus and concentrate on what was being asked of me. A welcome diversion. An opportunity for growth. Admittedly, it was not easy.

A new development started that week as well. My hair began to fall out. In fistfuls and handfuls, particularly in the shower: if I ran my fingers through my hair, between each digit would be long strands of hair. I wasn't horrified but amazed. I knew that this would happen, and there wasn't much I could do. I was going to be the rule, not the exception.

Tuesday arrived and as I got into my limo to head to *Canada AM*, the *Globe and Mail* was on the back seat. John, my driver, was like a proud father as he watched my reaction. There on the front page, across the top, was a full banner with a colour photo announcing my arrival to the newspaper. I was shocked, stunned. Who knew that the *Globe* would put a full banner across the front page? There I was, page A19, my words in a column that would last in perpetuity in the archives, not evaporate as I imagined my television appearances doing. I felt a little panicky. My first column was about how and why I had joined the paper. What if no one liked it? What if it came across as too self-indulgent? This was me, as vulnerable as it gets.

I did my segment on *Canada AM* and Seamus O'Reagan showed the paper on air, as my segment began, joking that I hadn't had enough to do before. I was embarrassed but admittedly proud. When I was finished with my segment, I finally read my column as it appeared in print:

My name is Dr. Marla Shapiro. Perhaps you know me from CTV simply as Dr. Marla. I am the medical contributor for Canada AM and I do regular medical segments for CTV Newsnet. On occasion, I appear on the National News with Lloyd Robertson doing my best to explain a current medical story. I also host my own weekday talk show called *Balance . . . television for living well.*

Until a few weeks ago, I ran a full-time Family Medical practice, seeing patients four or five days a week. People always ask me how I manage it all: a busy career or two, three kids and a husband, a household that rocks and rolls.

But all that seems easy compared to my newest task—being a patient. Which also leads me to how I started a new leg of my career, writing this column for The Globe and Mail.

I am excellent at juggling; it's how I keep my balance in life. I often give speeches about finding a HEALTHY balance, and talk about those familiar balls we all try to juggle—the "work" ball, the "family" ball, the "me" ball. While our hearts favour the family ball it seems that the work ball claims most of the hours of the day. As the so-called expert, I remind my audiences that it is easier to juggle two balls than three and even easier to juggle one at a time. We should give ourselves permission to concentrate on one task at a time and then, very mindfully, decide when it is time to put down that ball and pick up the others. It is one way to stop feeling so conflicted all the time, believing that we have to be in three places at once. You can only be in one place at a time, so decide where you want that to be and move along. It's a simple concept, but it does work.

The two balls most important to me are my family and my work. The "me" ball often gets shoved into a corner gathering dust. I promise to get around to that ball but there often are too many competing interests and not enough time.

On Friday, Aug. 13, I had a routine mammogram. That pointed out a suspicious area that ultimately led to the diagnosis of breast cancer. On that date, I joined a club that until then I had been the consultant for. Having a largely female practice, this is familiar territory: Diagnosing women, helping them sort through cancer treatment options, explaining that all cancer is not the same and helping them stay ahead of their anxiety is second nature to me. Suddenly, finding myself inside the examination room looking out rather than outside looking in, I realize that an important new voyage is about to begin for me.

Clearly, I do not want to define myself by my new diagnosis. As the e-mails and cards and letters have flooded in, I stare incredulously at the warm wishes for a speedy recovery. I certainly do not feel ill—and I keep wondering who they are talking about. Words like "sorry" get my back up and I reflexively remind people that they would have been sorry had the diagnosis been missed. The diagnosis has been made.

But if I take a step back, I understand what people, friends, family—all of them—are saying. Try as I might not to define myself by my breast cancer, it is clear that it is now dictating how I will spend the next several months.

I started chemotherapy three weeks ago, which will continue over the winter months. My particular chemotherapy regimen has me receiving the medication every two weeks. The rhythm of my life has now been defined by the anticipated side effects, the climb back up to feeling well, only to repeat the cycle again. White counts and neutrophils, lymphocytes— all fighter cells and the cornerstone of keeping germs at bay, plummet due to the toxic side effects of chemotherapy.

As a result, I cannot practice medicine, as my medical office that is my second home puts me at risk for too many infectious diseases as much of what I see are patients who are ill and contagious. I will still appear on Canada AM as I am able, and *Balance* will still air, but the profession that defines who I am has pushed me out of my second home. At least for the time being.

I have always seen medicine as a collaborative relationship between patient and health-care provider. Education is the basis of what I do: if my patients understand what motivates me to treat them the way I do, they are more likely to do it. Branching out into television was an opportunity to reach and teach more people about health matters.

So that brings me to this column, now part of my new "work" ball. The column will allow me to address your concerns as well as mine ranging from children, adolescents, women's and men's health issues and our aging demographic

So every two weeks, this is where you will find me. I hope that you will send me your questions and pick my brain. Of course, I cannot answer questions about your own specific health issues, which are between you and your doctor.

As the column title suggests, I am indeed "on call for your questions on issues of health and how to live well."

Well, if you'd missed the press release and the news statements on air three weeks earlier, you couldn't miss this. I had breast cancer. Welcome to my world. Now, I hoped, I could put it aside, at least in the column, and move forward.

I have always felt that luck is overrated. And I don't think I'm especially lucky. This column for the *Globe* was just one example from my career of using luck to my advantage. Luck is an opportunity that comes your way; chance is what you do with it—recognize the opportunity, take a chance and leap at it. This new writing endeavour made it clear to me that I was not going to be a victim. I had to make room to accommodate my cancer and respect what it dictated to me, but it would not dictate my entire life.

I also agreed to take on speaking engagements in the second week of my upcoming chemo treatments, as I could now see that I felt better and more functional during that second week.

By Thursday it was clear that my hair was falling out fast and furiously. I would take a shower and find myself standing in water up to my ankles as hair blocked the drain. I called my girlfriend Renee and we went to the hairdresser. For years my hairdresser had wanted to cut my hair; now I told her to cut it. She took me into a back room for privacy. I was somewhat surprised, since I didn't think it was necessary, but she told me that everyone would watch and this was as much for her as for me.

I asked her to cut off a few locks and as she did we tied four into bundles with red ribbons. Off came almost all my hair. I wasn't upset or shocked, but rather curious to see what I looked like with short hair. It was all right—in fact, kind of fun to have this new look. But within five minutes of leaving the shop, the national newsdesk at CTV called.

They wanted me to do a story that night on an outbreak of infection in a Quebec hospital. Of course I could cover the story, but I wasn't sure what to do about my hair—wig or no wig? I went in and did it with the new short hair. I got great reviews on the hair but I knew that the style was to be short-lived.

By the weekend, even the short hair was falling. It was all over the place. Again I called my hairdresser and she came over that Sunday and gave me a short, short haircut. Again I was amazed at how different I looked. It was a close-cropped little do, almost a buzz. But it felt liberating. I felt in control of what was happening—or at least deluded myself that I was in control.

Tuesday came, and another *Canada AM*: it was clear that I would have to wear the wig. It didn't make sense to have a buzz cut at 8 a.m. and be on air with *Balance* at 10 a.m. with long hair. The *Balance* shows were pre-taped but all new, and I didn't want viewers to think they were old. So on went "Judy," the Dr. Marla hair. I felt self-conscious and wondered if it looked like I was wearing a hat. I woke up Amanda at 5:45 a.m. to ask if I looked okay. Poor kid—half-asleep, she said I looked fine. I don't think she had really opened her eyes.

I walked onto the floor of the studio and Bev Thomson approached me. She asked how I was. She asked me if the hair was mine and I told her no, it wasn't. She immediately reassured me that it looked great and that no one would be able to tell. I wasn't sure I believed her, but will remain eternally grateful for the nod of approval just before air time. This was from a woman who had been there and done that and knew how difficult this really was. I put on a good show, but I was anxious.

That night, a girlfriend who is a stewardess dropped by. She told me that she was doing the Toronto–Tokyo flights and that she often visited a temple when she was in Japan. She asked me if I had something precious that she could have blessed for me. I had friends who asked rabbis to pray for me, friends who had made a prayer at the Wailing Wall, friends who lit candles for me. I was not sure what all these prayerful gestures meant, or who benefited more, the friend who made the offer or me, but who was I to knock any of it? I gave her a lock of my hair. It couldn't hurt!

I also gave each of my girls a lock of my hair. I am not sure what motivated me to do that. I had kept locks from each of their first haircuts. Losing my hair felt as though I was crossing a threshold into a future that would leave us all changed forever. It was as if this hair was my first haircut too.

TEN

Decisions and uncertainty

You might have thought that with many weeks of chemotherapy still ahead of me, I was exempt, for a time, from having to make decisions. No such luck.

The same day as my wig made its first appearance, I got an e-mail from Dr. Susan Love. Since I first told her of my diagnosis, she had been terrific in offering me her guidance. Now her input gave me yet more to consider about my own management, and again highlighted that there would be no single "right" answer here. She suggested that a double mastectomy might not be the route to go; radiation, she thought, might be better to deal with the lymphovascular invasion that was seen on my pathology report.

Dr. McCready too felt that with the lumpectomy done, I'd had all the surgical intervention necessary, and that radiation should be the next step. The recurrence rate was the same—10%—with either lumpectomy and radiation or with mastectomy. Even with a mastectomy, you can have recurrence in your chest. It is simply impossible to remove every single last cell. And I knew David wanted me to be clear that amputating my breasts was not his suggestion. But there was more to my concern than just the issue of recurrence. There was my real concern that I would never again be reassured by a mammogram, even in conjunction with MRI screening. Despite the fact that the mammogram had diagnosed me, a year earlier it had missed the cancer that was already there—cancer that likely was not invasive at that point.

My own oncologist, Dr. Trudeau, felt strongly that the two treatment options—breast conservation and radiation versus mastectomy—were equivalent. Both were likely to offer me the same long-term outcome, but knowing who I was as a person and as a physician, she recognized that I needed more information. She was arranging for me to get an opinion from a radiation oncologist, but that would not happen for another two weeks. I was prepared to wait. This was not an urgent decision, but it was a decision that needed to be made.

In the meantime, reading Dr. Love's advice, I was struck again by the fact that no decisions were black and white. As a doctor, I am asked all the time to make decisions for my patients. As a doctor who had now become a patient, I realized how difficult it was for me to believe that these decisions that we were trying to make about my mangement were the so-called right decisions. I recognized that these decisions were the best decisions that could be made in the light of present information. As a doctor, I could see the difference between the art and the science. Here was an expert with one point of view who differed from the expert who was taking care of me. So how to decide? Being me, it wasn't easy.

Shortly after this, I met with Andy Barrie, a friend and radio broadcaster on CBC's highly rated *Metro Morning* in Toronto. Over lunch he asked me an interesting question: was it better to be me, he wondered, and know as much as possible in making a decision, or was it better to know as much as possible about the people you allowed to make decisions for you? It was a great question that spoke to all the concerns I was having about the doctor as patient. I told him that for my entire adult life I had been a doctor and knew no other way, so I was doing my best to marry both sides of that question and be as reasonable as I could.

I refused to stay home and found myself at a large women's luncheon the next day. With my cropped do, I walked in knowing that I would be with more than 350 women, many of whom I knew as patients, friends or just individuals in the community. I braced myself for the inevitable, plentiful stares and comments. It was my first really large public outing following the *Globe and Mail* article and the short haircut. I could see women who were uncomfortable and didn't know what to say. Others came over to tell me they were thinking of me, or to comment on the article and the hair. Many wished me well.

Again—as with the e-mails and letters and phone calls—it was apparent that all the wishes, no matter how awkwardly some were phrased, came from the right place. I didn't find myself getting as angry as I might have before when someone would solicitously place her hand on my arm and say, "How are you? No, how are you *really*?" Again I found myself more upset by the women who turned away. *Cancer is not an infectious disease*, I wanted to scream. *I am fine*.

And so it went, the personal redefinition that was happening within me. I was still me, but somewhat altered, different. And if I could not put my finger on exactly what was different, I knew that a change was happening.

One person who had known the real me for many years—and who did not turn away when she heard of my cancer diagnosis—was a remarkable woman named Gwen Vineberg. When I was 12 years old, Gwen had been my grade 7 teacher, and she became my first true mentor, the person who taught me to think outside the box. She challenged me to read books about apartheid, develop a social conscience and think critically and honestly about difficult social and moral issues. She challenged me to believe that I could be anyone I chose to be, do anything I chose to do. She taught me that the greatest gift was striving for your dreams. I can still remember her—a tall, elegant woman standing at the chalkboard, imposing quiet on a noisy classroom in seconds by tapping the wide gold wedding band that she wore (and still wears). She commanded respect. I interviewed Dr. Phil a few years ago when he published *Self Matters,* and he talked about critical choices, defining moments and pivotal people. Gwen was one such pivotal person in my life, and she would set me on a path that would define who I have become.

Gwen and I became friends and have stayed friends all these years. When I first started practising medicine here in Toronto, she was diagnosed with stage 4 ovarian cancer—a poor prognosis with death almost a certain outcome. In those days there was no ondansetron to deal with nausea. I flew into Montreal to be with her for one of her chemotherapies. They kept you in hospital for chemo in those days. Gwen looked awful, near death even, but this woman was and is a fighter. It is no surprise that Gwen the educator survived her cancer and became a loud voice for women in their fight with ovarian cancer. In many ways she changed the way in which ovarian cancer has been dealt with in Montreal.

When my press release came out, Gwen immediately contacted me and wanted to know my chemotherapy schedule. On the Monday before my third session with AC, she took the train to Toronto. In her early 70s, she is still an impressive figure, stately and modern in her appearance. Always informed about most things, she is wonderful to talk to. I picked her up at the train. She cut a dashing figure in a beautiful orange leather jacket. That jacket would garner comments everywhere we went over the next 24 hours.

I wanted my friends to know this woman who means so much to me. So that evening I invited 15 women over for what I called a board of directors meeting, to meet the original CEO. Each of my friends brought something and in no time a gourmet feast was created. It was wonderful for me to see everyone interact and to hear them say that I "made cancer fun." I can't say that is really true, but it is true that I was determined not to let cancer keep me from enjoying the world I had created for myself since moving to Toronto. When I first arrived here to be with Bobby, I didn't know another soul, and I felt lonely, even desperate. I had lived in Montreal all my life, and while I loved Bobby, I missed the familiarity of my roots. That is likely why I continued in a residency training program, doing a concurrent master's degree; it gave me no time to acknowledge my loneliness. Now, some 23 years later, I was surrounded by friends who are as close as sisters, many displaced from Montreal and who therefore understood even more deeply how important we were and are to each other. The fun and camaraderie of that evening took me away, for a time, from all that was happening. Gwen gave me a copy of a book called *You Are Not Alone*, for which she was one of the contributors. She had inscribed it personally to me. Indeed I did not feel alone at that moment.

The next morning we awoke early and I took Gwen with me to CTV to show her how *Canada AM* and Newsnet were done. Nothing gave me greater pleasure than to show Gwen part of my world, a world whose doors she had, in so many ways, opened for me by pushing me to excel. I was proud and she, in turn, was proud for me.

When we got home and I took off my turtleneck, a large amount of my hair came with it. My housekeeper, Grace, noted that it was impossible to clean up these hairs; she had to pull the shorter ones out of my clothes because they would not wash out. I had also begun to work out again with Stacy, my trainer, and found loads of hair on the mat every time I did exercises on my back. Initially I thought it was dirt, but no, it was my hair.

Gwen gently told me that while my hair was *on* my head it was no longer *in* my head. A large bald patch had appeared on the back of my head from the rubbing that happened every time I lay down. I had been told that I would feel a tingling sensation in my head as the hair was getting ready to fall out. In fact I had been noticed tingling and a kind of contracting feeling in my scalp for the past week, but had studiously ignored it.

I don't think it coincidental that Gwen was with me, nor at the same time do I believe in divine intervention, but it was comforting to have her there, a woman who understood all of this so well, a woman who had beat the odds. Together we went out to the garage and I leaned over the garbage can. Gently, and without much effort, we rubbed my scalp and almost every strand of hair came out. Painlessly, swiftly, shockingly fast—out.

Gwen cut some of the longer residual strands and then I cautiously looked at my image—first, in the oven door so it would be somewhat distorted. Curious, I moved on to a mirror and was astounded to see my completely bald head. I called Grace to let her see as well; my housekeeper, without skipping a beat, smiled and said all I needed was earrings.

Gwen and I were picked up by Susan, who was joining us for lunch before chemo. I was wearing a short wig. At the restaurant, my still-sensitive appetite was in evidence: I could barely swallow the egg-white omelette I had ordered. It seemed the only foods I could handle these days were clear soups or egg-white omelettes. Not much else looked appealing—or stayed down.

Gwen gave the oncology unit a second copy of her book. She sat with me as my portacath was pierced and the drugs administered. I had a new chemo nurse this time, Claire. Having previously been a chemo nurse in a pediatric centre, she was warm and caring. She offered me a Popsicle to help get rid of the metallic taste that occurred during chemo and we joked that it had taken three sessions for me to get the Popsicle. We talked about the incredible constipation I was suffering, a common side effect, and she warned me of the danger of a peri-anal abscess. I was having a hard time getting bran and roughage down, which were former staples of my diet. Claire made the recommendation that I start some stool softeners and gave me an information sheet.

Buoyed by her frank approach, I asked her to talk to me about Taxol. I knew I was getting ahead of myself—it would be many weeks yet before I had to receive the four Taxol treatments—but I was curious and concerned. I had read the medical literature, but by now I realized that reading about and experiencing are eons apart. Claire told me that the Taxol would make me lose my eyebrows, which is tough because eyebrows frame the face. I made a mental note to call one of the CTV makeup people to order eyebrow stencils for me. For those without these contacts—that is, most people—the "Look Good, Feel Better" programs affiliated with oncology units are a must. Wigs, eyebrows—these are not frivolous. Losing your identity to a change in your physical appearance can be devastating, and caring for your appearance is therefore as much a part of wellness as taking your medications.

We finished the chemo run and Gwen had to leave for the train station. I was glad she had been with me for this transition in my physical appearance. Andrea, another close friend, came to sit for the last part of the session while I got my take-home drugs: Neupogen, dexamethasone, ondansetron, Nexium (my gut was in an uproar and my oncologist suspected erosive gastritis, a pre-ulcerous condition that would explain why I couldn't eat or digest), domperidone to chase the ondansetron/dexamethasone combo used for the first few days of nausea, lorazepam as a mild sedative to help combat the insomnia side effect of dexamethasone, Colace as a stool softener, and also milk of magnesia, glycerin suppositories and mouth rinses. Apart from the incredible cost of all these items, I could not get over how much support I needed in the form of medication.

I went home, feeling a little unwell. I took off the wig and was astounded at how cold my head felt. I simply was not prepared for this, and put on a baseball cap for a little warmth. Matt came home from religious school. He had been forewarned by Grace that my hair was all gone, but she told him I was still beautiful. As he came in the house, without so much as looking at me, he told me not to remove the baseball cap, that I looked scary. Amanda came in and looked at me and told me I looked fine. She went to do her homework.

I went to my study and Jenna happened to call from London. At the sound of her voice, I fell apart. This was the last thing I wanted—to be crying like this, with Jenna so far away and crying now too, worried about me. I tried to explain why I was weeping. No matter how clever I had been in cutting my hair in stages—a recommendation made to me by other cancer patients and by my nurses—I, like anyone, was just not prepared for how this felt. I tried to explain that it was really less about vanity than about what this said to me. The baldness told me I had cancer and that perhaps it could kill me. It is not that I had lived in a state of denial about my cancer, but this was sending me a very clear message. Looking at that bald and now vulnerable-looking woman in the mirror was perhaps the hardest thing to accept, the toughest hurdle to get over. Bev Thomson, host of *Canada AM*, experienced her hair loss differently. She once told me that when her last strand of hair had fallen out she went to the mirror and thought, I am still me. But I knew that I was not still me and I never would be again.

Like that invisible boundary I had crossed when my son Jason died, that boundary that separated my life into a before and after, this too was a before and after. I was not the same woman I had been before all this started. That is not to say I am either better or worse—but I am different. Many cancer patients have told me they would not wish this experience on anyone, but that the person who emerges from cancer is not the one who entered, and that if you allow it, another sense of self comes into focus. I was beginning to understand what they meant.

ELEVEN

Support—whether you want it or not

Chemotherapy began to further widen the things that I was perceived as being the expert on. Since those gruelling days of chemotherapy, many people have asked me what they can do to support someone—usually a friend or family member—who is going through this. I have some answers, but my answers of course come from my own experience—my experience of being someone who hates to ask for or accept help. People like me need some help to accept help.

Many people adapt well to the sick role. They clearly know what they can and cannot do and don't find it difficult to ask for help. Perhaps they are better communicators. There are all kinds of books written on the sick role and some of the secondary benefits one can gain. For me, no matter how I looked at it, there was no secondary gain, only the further frustration of not being able to do what I wanted or needed to do. It eventually became clearer to me that I did not have to do everything myself. And, surprise of surprises (I say that sarcastically), everyone does it just as well without me!

As the weeks of chemotherapy passed, I indeed had great

support at home from my husband and children, but I could not relinquish the stupid thought that I needed to do it all alone. They were pleased by the fact that I was now around the house so much more, yet I saw myself as "being underfoot." I was desperate not to change their lives, and wanted them to carry on with their activities as they always had. This was my issue, a constant internal struggle for me, and certainly not theirs—they were concerned and wanted to help in any way they could. I couldn't stand being perceived as helpless and eventually had to admit that I was the only one who saw me that way. While I knew that cancer was not only my disease, but the entire family's, I wanted to pretend that I could shield them, that their lives would be unchanged. Jenna and Amanda had been changed by the experience of losing a brother; it has always been clear to me that having suffered such a loss so young, they are more empathic and compassionate people. I did not feel they had more life lessons to learn from my cancer. These concerns, and my innate independence, combined to make it a struggle to accept any kind of help.

Reality, however, is a great leveller. Bobby works an hour out of Toronto, Amanda was in her graduating year of high school, Jenna was living two hours away and Matt was still only nine. They could not be there for me—physically—all the time. And though I persisted in believing that I could manage without any help, sometimes, in the days after chemo, it was impossible. Even worse, it was impossible for me to admit it.

But there were friends who got that about me and were smart enough to stop asking. First, there were my two sisters-in-law. Wendy lives close by and has always been there whenever needed. Jenna and Amanda are exactly the same age as her two boys and shared many activities together growing up; the four were more like siblings than cousins. Sandy lives farther away, and we had not been as close. She was on sabbatical from teaching during this time and would always take the time to show up with a tea or a latte, when I could stomach the latter, and just keep me company, passing the time together. A gift in the cancer was that Sandy and I became good friends. For that I am very grateful.

And my friends . . . friends showed up with soups or dinner, dropped by to take in the dry cleaning or called when they were at the grocery store. I would always say no, but they would push and remind me that if I didn't tell them what I needed, they would have to guess, and what a pain that was for them. They were relentless in their support as they began to understand the rhythm of the bad weeks. They would show up for car pool when Matt needed a ride to his afternoon program. I was ready to provide a car and driving lessons to a nine-year-old, but I didn't relish the idea of going to jail.

Then there was the kindness of virtual strangers. Bonnie Stern—an internationally known and acclaimed chef—had been on the show a few times. Bonnie started e-mailing me regularly to find out what I loved to eat and what I couldn't eat, and each week she would send me a menu that she thought might work. Without my asking—in fact, with my telling her it was not okay, that she should not do this—a meal would show up, delivered by cab and still piping hot. The truth is that I was constantly shocked by how chemo had changed what I could eat. Coffee—gone. Salads—gone. Even my guilty pleasure of chocolate almonds—gone. Each week, Bonnie would work hard to find something nutritious and easily digestible. Warmed roasted cauliflower soup became a favourite, bocconcini salad worked on occasion, apple crisp on a good week filled the house with incredible aromas. There were egg-white-and-spinach frittatas, grain salads, roasted vegetables. She tried endless options. And when it was clear I could not eat, she made cookies for the kids and other treats they might like.

I could not believe Bonnie's empathy and kindness. The night I came home hairless, devastated and overwhelmed, I found her food waiting for me. I wrote Bonnie a letter that very evening. Both the food she had sent and the gesture itself were so meaningful. Food sustains and nourishes, and though in receiving food from Bonnie I felt inadequate—it made clear that I could not always provide lovingly prepared meals for my family—I was also reminded of the nourishment that friends can offer if you allow yourself to take it. As I wrote to Bonnie, I felt relieved by this opportunity to talk about how I was really feeling. In part, here is what I wrote:

> I am not sure about the "why" of all your kindness other than to accept that you are so wonderful and giving. I have a hard time asking for anything, having lived my life as a doer, organizer and in-charge kind of person. . . . To find your kindness, the TLC that goes into your creations, the timing of it arriving to coincide with my getting home, and the soup and cake still being warm . . . it did me in. But did me in—in a good way.

> Bonnie, you just get it and I guess you get me. I can never repay your kindness, your thoughtfulness and [express] my gratitude in finding you in my life. What goes around comes around, or so they say. So you, my dear, have a lot coming.

Bonnie, you have touched me so deeply. You are indeed
a rare breed. If there is any silver lining in any of this,
then you are indeed a large part of that lining.
Thank you is inadequate.

Love, your very vulnerable and grateful friend . . . and I
do not use that word friend lightly.

Awestruck,
Marla

Bonnie's response was pure Bonnie, pure self-effacing
Bonnie. Simply put, she said that she liked to nourish, and
reminded me about the goodness of people, and the depth of
friendships and caring. But I knew she was nourishing far more
than just my body. A woman who had been a virtual stranger
had touched me so profoundly.

My girlfriend Lisa's husband, Phil, would e-mail me every
Thursday about his two-for-one special on foot massages. He
would take the time to find a great foot cream and show up
with it in hand, ready to go to work. He would catch me up
on his life while massaging my feet, and eventually, relaxed,
I would fall asleep. It amazed me that this busy lawyer and
friend would do this. At first it seemed so silly and frivolous, and we laughed about it endlessly, but it was a slice of
heaven, and I began to look forward to Thursday afternoons
as my "Phil time." And I thanked Lisa for her generosity in
sharing him.

Cards and letters from *Globe and Mail* readers continued to
come in, cards from patients, gifts. I was told that I was irre-
pressible, had fortitude. Children told me they were praying

for me. So much attention was embarrassing but heartwarming. It reminded me that everyone wanted to help.

From a patient:

I just wanted you to know that I think about you every day and know that all is going well. I have always admired your inner strength, optimism and positive thinking. YOU ARE MY HERO.

I know it's strange to say, but I miss you terribly, not knowing that I can get to see you when I need to, and it was always reassuring to know that I could pick up the phone and speak to you or see you.

Just wishing you the best and can't wait to see you in June 2005.

Her letter echoed many of my own thoughts. It was difficult for me to get up each morning and not get dressed and head to the office. I was not, for a time, a practising doctor and I was struggling without the identity that had defined me for so many years.

Some of the cards made me laugh, actually flat-out laugh. I loved the funny ones, the ones that didn't use the words *sympathy, ill, sickness* and the like.

One letter arrived with the heading, "Yes Dr. Marla, the Kvoleks have received their Flu Shot." Inside, each line funnier than the last, these patients reminded me how lucky I was. Their letter read:

Hello Marla,

Dan and I just want you to know that we suspect Osama Bin Laden is responsible for the War on Breast Cancer! The Bush

Administration was searching for the wrong weapons of mass destruction!

The "evil doers" have no idea who they are dealing with. Have they not seen your television show? Have they not had a physical, complete with Marla-esque blunt commentary? Have they not had a sneak attack flu shot? Have they ever tried to get past Rose [my other very competent secretary]?

As a family, our commitment to your well being will be to sustain ideal body mass, eat a diet rich in nutrients, manage our response to stress as best we can, and be active for 30 minutes each day. Of course, we will stray from the path from time to time and fall prey to the occasional Krispy Kreme. We may drink four instead of eight glasses of water a day. But as God is our witness, we will wear our seat belts, remain smoke free and use an SPF of 30 of higher.

Rise up, Marla. Sing Oh Canada in both official languages and take time to visit Bayview Village [a local shopping haunt].

[Signed by the Kvoleks]

As I read, I broke into gales of laughter. I had not heard myself laugh out loud in a while and it reminded me that indeed, as the saying has it, laughter can be the best medicine. It is a wonderful way to support someone.

Admittedly, there was nothing funny about the diagnosis of breast cancer. But as I struggled to define the new me and what I would do with all this time, I began to discover "retail therapy." Suddenly, with so much time on my hands when I felt well, I could peruse the stores. Bobby does all his banking online. He is an up-to-the minute credit card tracker and so he can joke that he always knows where I am, at any time and in any country! One day Bobby looked up at me and said, "Good news, bad news: you are going to survive the breast cancer. I, on the other hand, will be bankrupt." Later, when I met with Dr. Lipa to discuss the implants, Bobby came with me and asked if he had a say in size and was there anywhere he could take a test drive? While I think his joking question startled Dr. Lipa, I laughed, knowing that Bobby was doing his best to make light of a serious moment (and actually, it *was* funny). And so, with my own Bobby reminding me not to lose my sardonic edge, I tried to keep the laughs coming. We had to find—and keep finding—the humour in this situation.

My dear friend Dr. Robert Buckman was key in reminding me that laughter is therapeutic. Rob has appeared many times with me on *Balance,* his biting sense of humour and range of knowledge making him a constantly challenging sparring partner.

When he learned of my diagnosis, he was the first to send me a series of what he called "e-hugs," funny little e-mails reminding me to stay grounded and not to lose my sense of humour. I asked Robert if humour could be helpful in a strictly clinical sense, and he offered me a few slightly serious words about humour.

It's often said that there are some things you must never joke about—and anything to do with cancer seems to be one of those things. Well, with some trepidation—and with genuine acknowledgement of the need for sensitivity, taste and timing—I beg to differ.

I would like to suggest that a few small doses of humour at the right time and in the right context help you cope.

Let me explain.

What Humour Does for Us

When we laugh (and perhaps even when we merely smile, provided it is a deep and genuine smile!) we feel better. We don't know precisely why, but the current theory is that laughter increases the release of endorphins (inbuilt analgesic—pain-killers— manufactured inside the brain) and by this and probably by other means as well, laughter reduces the intensity of pain or discomfort and increases the sense of well-being.

I imagine that everybody knows that anyway. When you have some pain (a headache or a sore back) if you happen to get deeply involved with a comedy on TV or a funny film, for a period of time your pain shifts to the background a bit. There was even a time when it was widely held—and partly believed—that laughter might actually affect the outcome of a disease process. This followed in the wake of a book by Norman Cousins called Anatomy of an Illness, in which he felt that he had changed the outcome of his ankylosing spondylitis by intensive "humour therapy" involving him watching funny films and videotapes, all day, every day, for several weeks. Despite quite a lot of interest, there has been no hard evidence that this approach actually changes the progress of any disease—but even so it makes people feel better.

Psychologically, I believe that humour does several things for the person who makes the joke—I'll call her or him the "joker"—and for the person hearing or seeing it (can we coin a new word and call the recipient the "jokee"?).

I think of humour as a deliberate and knowing deviation from an expected sequence—so if the recipient is expecting to hear . . . a logical and accepted sequence—1–2–3–4, for example, then he or she might be amused if the joker takes a side-step and says the equivalent of 1–2–3-cucumber (although I do realize that isn't a particularly funny joke in itself).

A typical example (in print) is this well-known aphorism: "If a man speaks alone in a forest, and there is no woman there to hear him—is he still wrong?" The expected sequence—based on "if a tree falls in a forest and there is no one to hear it, does it make a sound?"—would, we imagine, end up saying something thoughtful and weighty. The "is he still wrong?" ending is unexpected, it is pointedly mocking of men and it is therefore politically correct as well. All of which add up to it being an acceptable joke.

By that means, then, humour helps the joker draw a frame around the subject (basically saying "you were expecting me to respond in X fashion, I am responding deliberately in Y fashion"). This is why humour is so useful as a coping strategy in dealing with a threat— it shows the jokee that the joker can see beyond the threat itself. This also explains why so many jokes are about subjects that are actually quite threatening in themselves and are certainly not intrinsically funny. For example, a vast number of current jokes are about airline travel, illness, sexual problems, disputes with in-laws, or financial woes—none of which are intrinsically amusing in themselves.

Hence a touch of humour by someone with an illness shows the jokees that she or he (the joker) is able to see around the threat—is able to draw a frame around it and partly cope with it. Furthermore, that touch of humour—because it underlines the expectations that are shared between the joker and the jokee—draws the members of the circle closer together. It strengthens the bond between the joker and the jokee.

Three Practical Guidelines for the Safe Use of Humour

In my view, then, humour is a very useful coping strategy, but there are three basic rules that you should always bear in mind. (They're like the warnings printed on take-out coffee cups that tell you that the coffee may be hot.)

First, not everyone has a sense of humour. If a person has not been known to use humour in the past, they are not likely to use it now when they are facing a threat.

Second, humour cannot be "inflicted. " You can't make a person change their mood by forcing humour on to them. If they are open to humour, it will work: if they are not open to it, it will fail. Third, you can only ever use humour after you have shown that you take seriously the serious matters. You can't use it before taking the serious issues seriously or instead of doing that. Humour is a reinforcement of the relationship between the joker and jokee—it can't create that relationship out of nothing.

So, if you are a patient with cancer, go ahead and try humour if you feel like it, after you've talked about the serious stuff. And if you are a friend or family member, try a touch of humour IF the patient is the kind of person for whom humour has been useful in the past and AFTER you have shown that you are capable of taking the serious stuff seriously.

With those three main principles (or cautions) you should be all right. Perhaps the best evidence comes from what a patient told me about her own breast cancer. She had had a mastectomy about twenty years previously and had an external prosthesis (a "falsie" as she called it) which she wore under her clothing. It fell out of her bathing costume while she was swimming laps with a friend, who hissed at her "Doris, your THINGY has fallen out!" She told me that her response was to look at it floating away towards the shallow end and simply say, "Oh, there it goes—doing the breast stroke on its own."

Now THAT is a coping strategy.

And so, there are some words of wisdom from my friend Rob Buckman, who came around as often as I would let him for a cup of tea and an e-hug delivered in person.

The night that Bobby rolled over and said, "Put on your cap, the glare from the clock off your head is keeping me up," I actually laughed out loud. And realized, with relief, that my sense of humour was still intact.

TWELVE

Janice, Judy—and the bald eagle

After some 20 years of caring for all kinds of patients, the boundary between doctor and patient can get blurry. While I always tell my patients it is an inequitable relationship—I know everything about them while they know much less about me—there are times when my personal life will creep into my practice, and vice versa. Try as I might not to get involved in the emotional aspects of caring for my patients, I suffered personally along with their losses, their diagnoses that I could not cure, and personal events that left them unhappy and shattered.

Now, with the publicity surrounding my diagnosis, many of my breast cancer patients wrote to tell me how they had coped, the words of comfort I had given them. They reminded me that now it was time to draw on those words for myself.

One patient, who had suffered bilateral malignancies and had aggressively fought back with chemo, surgery and all the other options presented to her, showed up to remind me that we had yet to celebrate her progress. Along with her she brought her wig, a cute cropped version of what she looked like prior to losing her hair. Her hair had grown back and her wig had been relegated to a box, which she now brought over to my home. I called the wig, like her owner, Janice. Janice told me that she was a party wig, meant to go out and live life and not meant to be a cover-up of a tragic circumstance. The words echoed in my head, as I was sure I had used them myself before. So on my head went Janice, an easy-to-wear little wig that kept my head warm as the days got colder. My own wig, which we had named Judy for the lovely woman who had crafted it, had now assumed the nickname of Dr. Marla, and I seemed to reserve her for television appearances, as it was so close to the hair I had prior to losing it all.

At first I saw these wigs as my closest friends, links to my previous reality and who I was. I wore the wigs everywhere, whether I was running errands or appearing on television. At home, I never wore a wig, feeling entirely comfortable as long as I was warm. You could usually find me in either my trusty red cap, which made me look like one of the seven dwarves, or my black yoga cap. But something interesting happened—and I am not sure why or how it did.

One Saturday evening, on a weekend before a chemo, a weekend that would invariably find me in my best shape, Bobby and I got ready to go out to see friends. It was one of my few social forays in a while. As I descended the stairs, he stopped me and asked if I had forgotten something. I realized that I was walking out without my wig. The kids—including Matt, who had at first been so afraid to see me bald—had gotten used to my shiny head; it was becoming part of the landscape of our home. When I ventured to peer in the mirror, I was beginning to realize that this bald-headed version of Marla who looked curiously back at me was, in fact, me. The wig that was Dr. Marla began to make me realize that I was more than just Dr. Marla. The ability to "put Dr. Marla in a box" began to feel appealing. Maybe I could put Dr. Marla in a box altogether and let Marla out.

Although I wore the wig out that night, the thought began to pull at me: what would happen if I didn't? What would I think, what would other people think? With my growing acceptance of my hairless appearance, I began to wonder if the wig was more for other people's comfort than my own. I was becoming more comfortable in my new reality than pretending that I lived in my old reality.

That Tuesday, when I went in to *Canada AM,* I brought the wig in the box and had the make-up people put on my "television face" bald-headed. Not only was it easier to put on the makeup without fear of getting it all over the wig, it was entirely more comfortable. The first few times we did makeup this way I got odd stares and comments but was quick to laugh about it. It was odd that some people did not recognize me. The president of the network did a double-take, not quite placing me without my hair. While it was clear that I would always appear on air with the Dr. Marla wig, I was beginning to feel more comfortable without it.

The Women in Film and Television Awards luncheon was the first place that I chose to go wigless. Kim Cattrall was the guest of honour. It was somewhat ironic, given that she had played a breast cancer patient on *Sex and the City.* She and I were photographed together as some media outlets saw the irony of the two of us together. While indeed I did garner a few odd stares, I felt mostly comfortable with my new bald status. Here, among people who I worked with, there was the attempt not to show shock or disapproval on their part, but I felt somewhat defiant. Cancer is not only something you talk about. You actually can look at it too.

My parents came to visit, taking the train in from Montreal. Both are well into their 80s and this was not a physically or emotionally easy trip for them. I imagine they must have rehearsed their response to my new look because, even before they'd actually looked at me, they told me I was beautiful. I chaired the Osteoporosis Society of Canada's Bone China Tea and my parents were my guests. I got ready to leave the house without the wig and my dad asked me where it was. He wasn't judging me, but rather being protective; he wanted to be sure I wouldn't be made fun of. I appreciated his warmth and caring but reminded him that this is what I truly looked like. People would get past it—and if not, then not. It would be their issue and not mine. So I appeared wigless in front of some 700 women. My parents sat proudly in the audience and were thrilled when the Osteoporosis Society acknowledged me for my volunteer work with them. My mother focused more on the work I was doing and began to no longer see her bald daughter.

The Geminis were next and I had been nominated for a Viewer's Choice Award. Wigless I went. People thought I was brave and courageous but that really had nothing to do with it at all. I wasn't trying to make a bold statement or become the poster child for women with breast cancer. There was no statement other than "This is what women with cancer look like." I was simply living in my own reality, and bald was part of it.

I did get some odd comments, particularly at the Geminis, that were stupid. Some people thought I was trying to make a statement and draw attention to myself, but they were mostly unaware of my breast cancer. Those who were aware simply wished me well. It did make it back to me, however, that some of my friends—not the close ones, but acquaintances rather than friends—thought it was disgusting that I was "prancing around bald." Believe me, there was no prancing. There was slow, let-me-get-through-this-day walking. Experiences like these have the effect of separating the real friends from those who simply love to gossip. I was learning that those who judged were laughable. I wasn't sure what gave them the authority to judge me and know what was best, but I did my best to ignore the comments that I heard and tried not to be hurt in the process. I was amazed that I was not angry. The anger was beginning to dissipate and that was a very important sign of my beginning to accept what was happening to me.

Jenna's 20th birthday was in my final week of AC treatment. That treatment proved to be incredibly difficult, with horrible fatigue and nausea. The feeling of being bathed in toxic waste left me unable to eat and uncomfortable in my own skin. But we were determined to drive up to her university as a family so that we could take her out to dinner and celebrate with her. I did my best to sleep during the two-hour drive but the nausea and feeling of unwellness were so pervasive I was afraid I wouldn't make it. But eventually we did get there, and she was thrilled to have us with her.

In many ways, with Jenna away at school, she was limited in her ability to support and in turn be supported. There was no one to answer her fears when she called and I sounded unwell, or when she called and I was resting, something that in all her 20 years she had never really seen. But we made it through the day and went out for dinner and had her friends back to her little house. They all got their first look at me wigless and commented on what a great-shaped head I had. As we brought out the cake and Jenna made her wish, it was painfully obvious to me what she was wishing. It seemed unfair that she should have to make a wish about me; this should have been entirely

"Jenna time" as she moved out of her teens and entered adulthood. As she finished making her wish and got ready to blow out her candles, I looked at her and whispered, "I will be," and we both fell into a puddle of tears.

The day ended with hugs and kisses and both of us wondering if I would always be there with her to celebrate, neither one of us giving voice to our fears. I realized that we stood at a doorway that she was about to go through, never to return. My children had lost their innocence about our ability to protect them and always be there for them, and she had turned a corner into adulthood. Along with her siblings, even Matt, she was being rushed into a reality from which I had hoped to spare them.

THIRTEEN

Enter Taxol

As I finished my fourth and final Adriamycin/Cytoxan treatment, I was unwell. I had trouble eating and now my hemoglobin had fallen from a normal of 138 to 82, which is frighteningly low. I found it difficult to breathe, had trouble going up the stairs without stopping and felt light-headed in the shower. Dr. Trudeau and I talked about a blood transfusion but I refused. Realizing I could not suffer the risk of any more bone marrow toxicity, we agreed that I would start on Eprex, a synthetic version of epoetin alfa, which is produced naturally by the body but is often compromised in cancer patients. This was not an easy decision for me. I was fighting the addition of any more drugs, wanting to do this on my own. But it was clear I could not. I was getting too sick and eventually the shots seemed better than a transfusion.

The regimen being offered was a once-weekly 40,000-unit injection that I could administer at home along with the daily shots of Neupogen that I was already taking to maintain my white count. The weekly shot was meant to maintain my hemoglobin and improve the quality of my life, which had been rapidly deteriorating with the dose-dense regimen. It was also meant to reduce the necessity for transfusion.

It can't be easy to have me as a patient. At that visit I mentioned that I had noticed a small mass in my right breast, the side with the cancer. It felt firm and cyst-like and I pointed it out to Dr. Trudeau. She agreed that I could have an ultrasound and if it was cystic we would aspirate it. This is a procedure she doesn't do. Being a family doctor, I actually often do aspirations. I asked her for a syringe and, with my girlfriend sitting there, under appropriate sterile conditions, I actually aspirated my own lesion. Dr. Trudeau had a lot to put up with.

And then there was the knowledge factor: I was aware of almost every possible side effect. Dr. Trudeau knew how hard it was for me to simply be a patient and accept her advice. The question that Andy Barrie had asked me over lunch (was it better to know so much or better to accept advice from the best doctors) kept coming back to haunt me. I realized I would have preferred to simply feel confident about my doctors' knowledge and expertise, rather than being me—who did not know nearly as much as my oncologist, but enough to worry about every little thing, from side effects to my long-term prognosis. Indeed I did believe I had chosen the doctor who knew best and knew most, but it was hard to check my anxieties and queries at the door. Maureen seemed to know that about me and never gave me a hard time about all my concerns. It was to her credit that she realized I was not challenging her, but in the way that all patients need reassurance at different levels, this was the level of reassurance I needed. I admired her, her willingness to help me through this without once feeling threatened or getting the message that I doubted her expertise or authority. Dr. Trudeau gave me a review paper from the

Journal of Clinical Oncology so that I could feel more informed and more comfortable, and later I spoke to her about the option of the Eprex, which she was strongly pushing.

I had told her I was afraid of adverse outcomes for my red blood cells and, in anticipation of this discussion, she had highlighted sections from the medical journal article. I realized that I didn't even want to review the article. I truly did not want to be my own doctor. I wanted what she was giving me: acknowledgement that my concerns were real and had been weighed, but reassurance that this was still the best decision she could offer me.

With that, I took my first shot of Eprex and was sent to start the next of four chemotherapies.

I was fearful about starting Taxol. I knew it was likely that I would lose my eyebrows and lashes but I was more worried about the other side effects.

Because Taxol has such a high rate of adverse effects when first given, it is administered in a room with many patients where a nurse can monitor you closely. I was pre-medicated with a high-dose steroid and intravenous Benadryl to lessen the possibility of an adverse reaction. The Benadryl made my joints ache and made me feel immediately unwell. The nurse gave me a sublingual (under the tongue) Ativan despite my protests that I did not want to be sedated. The first Taxol is administered at an excruciatingly slow drip rate so that any early sign of reaction can be picked up. Every 10 minutes my blood pressure, temperature and oxygen saturation were measured. Nine hours later, I was sent home.

Taxol causes far less nausea than AC but it had the unexpected and very frightening reaction of giving me numbness in my hands and feet. I had painful tingling and discomfort—like frostbite—in my joints and hands that persisted for days. When I showered, the water felt too hot or too cold. It was too painful to type on the computer and I found wearing shoes impossible. I found myself paralyzed by my discomfort and the fear that it wouldn't go away. Worst of all, I found myself becoming increasingly despondent and socially isolated. I didn't want to speak to my friends. It was impossible to explain the discomfort and for the first time in a long time I felt angry at the world.

Months later, when I interviewed Melissa Etheridge, she would talk about Taxol. We had undergone the same treatment schedule. She talked openly about her decision to use medical marijuana rather than ondansetron to fight the nausea, and I could understand how much more appealing that might have been than dealing with the horrific constipation. She discontinued Taxol after the second round. This was understandable: if I was becoming despondent at the thought of not being able to work at a computer, how must the numbness and tingling in her fingers have made her feel? Music and the guitar are her very life. I forged ahead with the treatment but I was an emotional mess.

As I withdrew, my friends became distressed that I was not answering the phone. Some became upset with me. I angrily told them this wasn't about them, it was about me, and I wanted to be left alone. I wanted to feel sorry for myself. I didn't want them around me. I was constantly on the brink of tears and I began to wonder if I was getting depressed. I sat there enumerating my symptoms: inability to eat and sleep, loss of interest in things that usually excited me, anger, low sense of self-worth. Having ticked just about every symptom on the clinical depression checklist, was I now clinically depressed? Or was I perhaps entitled to feel this way without labelling myself with yet another disease?

Despite the way I felt and my new greenish skin colour, I continued to do *Canada AM*. Bev Thomson would later tell me that there were times she worried I should not be there. I was pushing too damn hard. My friends couldn't understand how, being so ill, I could go on air. It was impossible for me to explain that I hung on to this as my only sense of self, my only way of recognizing who I was. I was struggling to recover my self-worth.

It wasn't until day 10 that the symptoms, the dark haze of fear and depression, began to lift. With enormous relief I realized that the symptoms and side effects were unlikely to be permanent. But I was terrified that I had to endure three more treatments.

My son Matthew did his best to entertain me. I kept forgetting to give myself my shots and his actions let me know that, as much as I thought I had protected him from all the details, this amazing little boy knew so much more than I gave him credit for. On the Mondays before chemo he had learned to ask me what my counts were, knowing that a decent white count meant I could have my chemo and be one treatment closer to the end. He made a flow chart of when I was to take my Neupogen and he questioned me on when the new needle—the Eprex—was to be given. In elaborate detail he charted out schedules in different colours and posted them on the fridge. More than once, he reminded me to give myself an injection that I had forgotten about.

Cancer—not just my disease, but the whole family's. Whereas Matthew's initial concerns about my baldness and his friends had been so worrisome to him, they had completely melted away. He was used to seeing me bald and no longer thought it strange. He didn't seem concerned about the impact on his friends any longer and told them all we were in a war and we were beating cancer. I don't think it occurred to him that we might not win. To him, it was only a matter of time.

I continued to exercise along with the help of my trainer, who now came to the house. On the days I could barely breathe, Stacy pushed me to stretch and strengthen, and on the days I felt better, it was boot camp. Stacy in so many ways was responsible not only for my physical health but also my mental health. She had just had a baby, so there in the dead of winter she and her new baby would head over to my house to work with me. She brought me articles on the importance of exercise and wellness, and I promise you that she was right. Staying fit was my best defence. I could see how easy it would have been to crawl into bed and atrophy away, wither away. But no one was having any of that. I did my best not to pick up the phone and cancel, though it would have been so much easier to be alone. I was lucky enough to have Stacy to work with me, and I am eternally grateful to her. There are many fitness and wellness organizations attached to cancer treatment units. If you can have a friend drag you out to give your muscles a stretch, even when you feel that you can't, believe me that you can and you will be so much the better for it.

As my depression began to lift and I got ready for round two of Taxol, I began to read my e-mails again. From a friend, a professional, a man whom I certainly didn't credit as being emotional (okay, so I am biased in thinking that women are more in touch with the emotional side of themselves), I got this e-mail. I had sent my girlfriends a group mailing trying to explain why I had been so quiet, why this had been so difficult, and asking them to put up with me. I needed to get them off my back. Instead, this response came:

Dearest Marla,

I just read your mailing to the girls. There is a flip side. Jokes aside, it is so easy to talk and easy for me to say but you are living it . . . Think of all the people everyday that go through this shit without your strength and support. You have so much . . . firstly yourself and who and what you are, your ability to understand and step back from the moment to reflect to yourself and friends. The great family you have, Matty, the girls (what my wife would not give for a daughter) and Bobby, who even I would marry. It is like any other journey, the long paddle, the arms ache, there is no end and yet somehow we make it and the camp fire is warming. We make it through because there are others that are there for us and relying on us. We make it through because there is no choice. My thoughts are with you every moment of every day. While there is nothing I can say, there is knowing that you are not alone, in fact or in spirit. Take strength from those around you and look forward to tomorrow. We all wish there was more we could do, to be helpless is no salvation, but this time will pass and tomorrow will bring the memories for the future that will be full of fun, love and great times.

If there is anything let us know, we will do anything anytime.

love
Murray

He was right. Taxol might be telling me otherwise, but it was time to return to the land of the living.

FOURTEEN

Keeping it normal,
and the certainty of uncertainty

Around this time I heard again from Susan Love. Dr. Love had been wonderful in answering my questions, but it was clear that her approach was somewhat different than the approach of my own doctors. And here I need to stress again that in cancer there is no right answer. The "certainty of uncertainty" I call it. In the absence of knowing, there are clinical trials that your doctor looks at to best match your scenario with the treatment options out there.

I was beginning to weigh my next steps and was leaning towards a bilateral mastectomy. My radiologist had told me how difficult my mammograms were to read and there was no doubt that the previous year's mammogram, which had been read as normal, had cancer in it, likely at that point an innocuous ductal carcinoma in situ, but it had been missed because of my dense tissue. My own oncologist thought this was a reasonable approach and my geneticist, despite the fact that I was gene-negative, also thought this was a reasonable approach. Remember that in my non-cancerous side, the biopsy that I had insisted on through the painful MRI localization had shown a complete array of atypical ducts and cells that put me at risk for future cancer.

In my case—and I stress *in my case*—I had no confidence in the radiological tests available to me. I realized an MRI could "overcall" normal tissue and that technically doing MRI biopsies is difficult at best. With my dense breasts, I didn't trust the digital mammogram to be clear enough that results called normal would be truly normal.

I had seen Dr. Lipa, the reconstruction plastic surgeon, who thought this was a reasonable course. I had nursed patients through the painful and difficult multi-step reconstruction. I knew it would be painful and I knew it would not be easy. I also knew it would not be a guarantee. But at 48, I could not see myself worrying every six months about a diagnostic mammogram or MRI that would not, in any case, leave me completely reassured.

Dr. Love felt differently. My breast cancer had shown lymphovascular invasion. My nodes were negative but the invasion meant that there were early signs of spread, which of course was why we were doing the chemotherapy. She felt that radiation was a better choice. She felt that the chemotherapy would put me into menopause (hello—it had—welcome to my world of night sweats) and that being in menopause would reduce the risk on the so-called normal side by about 86%. That number was not high enough for me. She saw no advantage (and perhaps even disadvantage) to bilateral mastectomy. She got a smile of out me when she said that she would still sell me life insurance. Her viewpoint was that radiation would be a better answer than mastectomy and reminded me that recurrence following mastectomy was still in the range of 5 to 10%. I knew that Dr. Love had a point, but to me the 14% rate of possible disease on the left side was unacceptable. I asked to see a radiation oncologist to seek another opinion.

And so, the certainty of uncertainty. Is there really a right answer? There is no right answer. That was clear. And because each and every tumour has its own "fingerprint," what might be right for me (and who knew if indeed it was right?) might not be right for someone else. The public perception—that being "Dr. Marla" meant I was sailing through this with all the right answers—could not have been further from the truth. I was having trouble making decisions, just like anyone else. In fact, for me, this was torture.

I spoke with the radiation oncologist, and we reviewed all the data. There was concern that the margin closest to the skin was very small and that radiation wouldn't necessarily get that and mastectomy would. She felt that with the tumour load being moderate and the nodes being negative, radiation would be equivalent to mastectomy. She disagreed that mastectomy would not deal with the issue of local recurrence and, in light of my concerns, the bilateral mastectomy was a reasonable decision, one that she supported. Should there be any surprises in the final pathology when the breasts were removed, she said, we would have to talk about radiation. She encouraged me to go ahead with the two-step procedure of removal and initiating the reconstruction, since she felt the likelihood of residual disease was low. She pointed out, however, that should there be residual disease and the reconstruction had been done, there would be a 40% risk of contracture of the temporary capsule. I was willing to take that risk.

In addition, my friend and oncologist Dr. Robert Buckman spoke with a colleague at the M. D. Anderson Cancer Center at the University of Texas, who assured him there was nothing in the literature that either of us had missed. There were no studies suggesting that lymphovascular invasion meant that mastectomy and reconstruction were poor or inadequate treatment options.

For many of my patients, the thought of having a mastectomy is traumatic. Many people use the words *amputation* or *mutilation.* And for many of them and their partners there is significant concern about how mastectomy will change them physically, how it will affect their sex lives. Bobby trusted me to get all the medical opinions I needed. He was by my side when we listened to information from various specialists and it was clear that at times the talk was so clinical it was difficult for him to follow—much like it would be for me at one of his business meetings. But for Bobby, the discussion boiled down to one thing: it came down to life. All he cared about was me living. And while it was clear that mastectomy might not change the odds, it seemed that it would make me less anxious, and thereby improve the emotional quality of my life. He insisted it would not change anything between us, and again, with that typical sense of humour, he reminded me that there were great cosmetic surgeons out there and I would be new and improved. On a serious note, he supported me in every possible way to reassure me that this decision had nothing to do with the way I looked. It had to do with my being alive, being there, our being a family. He allowed me—and I tried to allow myself—to remove any of those concerns from the decision. I wasn't naive enough to think that it would not be difficult and would not affect the way I looked at myself, but for both Bobby and me that was the least of our worries.

With that, and understanding the certainty of uncertainty, I made my decision in consultation with my doctors and was determined not to revisit the decision again. Not surprisingly, it would turn out to be impossible not to look back, second-guess and revisit, but I was determined to make thoughtful decisions the first time around, understanding there was no turning back.

For women with breast cancer, there is indeed a leap of faith required. It is important to trust your doctor, understand there may not be a single right answer, and know that breast cancer is not one disease but a plethora of diseases. Any decision is made with your particular scenario in mind. My being a doctor did not mean my decision was any more right or ultimately better. But it was a decision made.

The last decision to consider was that of a hysterectomy. I was gene-negative and so, again, it was not essential. But I had met and spoken with the head of gynecology and gynecologic oncology at Princess Margaret Hospital, Dr. Joan Murphy. She agreed that my being gene-negative was something of a relief, not only for me but for my children. The decision to have the hysterectomy was more about the balance of risks than any overwhelming predisposition to malignancy. However, the removal of my ovaries would offer me some peace of mind. I was ER-positive, which meant that estrogen drove my tumour, and even during menopause the ovaries can put out estrogen. I realized that hysterectomy was an aggressive move, as did Dr. Murphy, but it was not unreasonable, and I had decided to be aggressive within reason.

Bobby and I met with Dr. Murphy for the last in a series of consultations about my surgical management. In considering the options, we knew the decision was mine. It was elective surgery, with many side effects, so I would not have it at the same time as the mastectomy and reconstruction. Dr. Murphy offered me two surgical dates. The first interfered with a golf trip Bobby had planned and so I generously offered to take the later date. But within five minutes, I looked at him and said, "No way. You can go golfing, but I'm taking the earlier date." Every minute seemed like an eternity and I was willing to do anything I could to get through this process. Bobby realized he would not be golfing, and I think Joan Murphy was waiting outside for me to change my mind to the earlier date—she understood I wanted this over. She joked that I had been generous of spirit in accepting the later date and I volleyed back, "Not that generous." We booked the surgery for nine weeks after the mastectomy and initial reconstruction. I wondered if I would ever see the light at the end of the tunnel.

Christmas break was approaching. As a family with crazy schedules we had always made a point of going away at Christmas. Over the past several years we had gone away with other families so that the kids, at their various ages, would always have others to hang out with and entertain themselves. This year we had planned to go with Bobby's brother and his wife (my dear friend Wendy) and two other families to the Caribbean. Now it became clear that I could not go. I had chemo scheduled over the New Year's week and I was not missing it. Furthermore, with my low white counts, air travel was not smart and the change in temperature from the frigid cold of Toronto to the heat of the Caribbean would not be wise.

Bobby didn't want to go without me. I insisted that he take the kids and go. It wasn't that I was a martyr, and I don't think I was consciously trying to teach them how life might be without me, but I wanted them to go—I wanted them to go on living. It was more of that ongoing struggle I had between "my" disease and "our" disease. I just couldn't see why they should stay home to watch me get sick from a Taxol run. My friends thought I was crazy and commented that surely Bobby and the kids would not go. But the more I thought about it, the more I felt that having them stay home made no sense. Jenna would be home from university. The three kids hardly spent time together as a unit and I knew they would if they were all away. I finally came up with a plan that seemed to make everybody happy. My sister, Zozzie, and brother-in-law, David, would fly to Toronto the day Bobby and the kids left. They would keep me company and take me to chemo, and I would have some "alone time" with my sister. She was only too happy to do it and knew she could fly if David was with her. Eventually I wore Bobby down, perhaps because the idea of taking his frustrations out on a golf ball really appealed to him. Matt was excited, but offered to stay home with me, as did each of the girls. The reality was that they were going.

A few weeks before Christmas we got a call that Lawrence, one of Bobby's closest friends, was unwell. Bobby has always amazed me with his ability to stay in touch with his friends, regardless of where they live. Weekly phone calls, visits—Bobby and his close friends are as supportive of each other as my closest girlfriends and I. Bobby and Lawrence had known each other since elementary school. Along with a handful of others, Lawrence was the glue that kept Bobby together after Jason died and after his father died. They shared years of history that cemented the bond between them.

Now we heard that Lawrence was fatigued and bloated and had abdominal pain. A series of tests showed that he had an intra-abdominal mass that looked large. It had all happened so suddenly, without much warning. I had a very bad feeling, that clinician's instinct that you can't explain but is born out of years of practice. The Sunday before Christmas, at my urging, Bobby flew to Montreal. Lawrence had been admitted to the emergency room of a Montreal hospital. Bobby was worried when he came home; Lawrence did not look well. Lawrence required urgent surgery to resect (cut out) the mass, which was more than likely a tumour. It reminded me that life is uncertain for all of us, even those of us without a diagnosis. At the onset of my illness Lawrence and his wife, Jeanette, had been so concerned, so supportive, and now suddenly he was far more ill than I was.

The morning of Christmas Eve a limousine arrived at 5 a.m., not to take me to work, but to take my family to the airport. I had been up the whole night with Amanda as she tweaked and finished all her university applications. Neither one of us had gone to bed. Finally, just before five, she took a shower and read-ied herself to go. I stood there at the door feeling as if I were watching them from afar, with a sense that if I died they would do this, the four of them, without me. I shook off the feeling, kissed them all and told them to get the heck out of there and get a suntan for me. As the door shut, I sat down on the stairs in disbelief—not that they had gone, but that I had this cancer that was keeping me from being part of my family. I fell into bed, exhausted from being up all night, and tried to sleep.

It wasn't long before Zozzie and David arrived. My friend Wendy, of CTV's *National News*, was also home alone for four days while her family was in Montreal. She would be working over the holidays, but we would all keep each other company. I had planned an elaborate Christmas Eve dinner, which was kind of odd since I had never done that before, but I wanted to have a festive atmosphere around the house. The four of us laughed through dinner.

Then Jeanette called. We had been exchanging phone calls all week, with me in the familiar role of doctor/adviser but also, and more important, friend. She told me that Lawrence had had his surgery to resect the tumour, it had gone well and he was in the intensive care unit. I was so grateful. After several tries I managed to get hold of Bobby and tell him the good news. He was elated and relieved.

Three short hours later, Jeanette called in a panic to say things had taken a turn for the worse. Then, within the hour, Lawrence died. I couldn't believe it, as much as I had feared it. I decided not to call Bobby back immediately, but to call him in the morning. There was nothing he could do from where he was. I knew that this loss would be terrible for Bobby, more of his world unravelling, and the distance would only punctuate that loss.

The next day I had planned a Christmas Day brunch. All the stores were closed and I had invited any friends who were around the city. Company dropped by all day; they took my mind off being without my kids and husband, and away from what Jeanette and her children must be going through. But I could not stop wondering how they were doing, how they were feeling, and imagining how terribly painful this was for them.

I had managed to plan an event for every day leading up to the chemo so that we wouldn't just sit around. Boxing Day we all went shopping, pushing our way through the crowds. It was freezing but we had a good time. We went to bed exhausted. At 3 a.m. the ringing phone woke me. It was Wendy, heading to work. Since she was alone I had asked her to let me know that she was fine and to call if she needed anything. Tsunami, she said. I had no clue what she was talking about until she explained that a tsunami had devastated parts of Southeast

Asia and was thought to have killed hundreds of thousands. Again I was struck by the uncertainty of life. Who could have foreseen or imagined the devastation that this act of nature, this force of nature, would wreak. Lawrence's loss, a devastating tsunami . . . Life was uncertain.

On Wednesday morning my sister and David took me to chemotherapy. Though I had an appointment, the doctor had forgotten to write the order, and I had to sit there pointlessly waiting for the on-call doctor to write the Taxol order. I was furious, agitated and impatient sitting and waiting hour after hour for the order to be written. It seemed so ironic that I had decided to stay in Toronto to complete the chemo and here there was no order written. By the two-hour mark, my regular chemo nurse called me in and started the pre-Taxol prep in an attempt to calm me down; the order would be there shortly. The pre-medication made me sick and achy. The dexamethasone made me feel mid-gut pain, as if I had an ulcer. Ranitidine, the intravenous meant to combat the pain, did nothing. The Benadryl drip given to preempt any allergic response made me feel cold. I had learned to bring my own blanket, and now my resolve had given way to accepting a milligram of lorazepam to sedate me so that I would sleep through it all. By mid-afternoon we were finally done and went home. I was feeling sleepy and unwell.

I went to sleep and David screened all calls, but I was touched that most of my friends on vacation called me from Mexico or Florida or wherever they might be.

On New Year's Eve at 9:30 p.m., my family got home, tanned and joyful. I was grumpy and unwell but glad to have them home. We went to a friend's home with a few other close couples to celebrate the New Year, with the obvious toast that 2005 should bring us all health. I barely stayed awake. Everything seemed arbitrary to me. This was just another night.

I was having terrible trouble sleeping. Between feeling unwell and the menopausal night sweats, which were horrendous, I could no longer sleep more than 30 minutes at a time. I was reluctant to take any medications so instead busied myself in the middle of the night with baking, laundry, researching stories and playing solitaire on the computer.

I was living my life in two-week stretches. The week of chemo, the daily shots so that I could expedite the chemo cycle to a 14-day run rather than the usual 21, and the week of beginning to feel a touch better—so that I could do it all again. Towards the end of the second week of a Taxol course, the now-familiar fiery sensation in my feet and hands would get a little better and I found that I could type at the computer or actually put on a pair of shoes. I was beginning to trust that I would not be left with a permanent neuropathy of numbness and burning, though the possibility still haunted my thoughts. If I lost sensation in my fingers I would have difficulty being a doctor; tactile sense is so important in examining a patient and making a diagnosis. The ability to feel subtle abnormalities while performing a breast exam . . . I shuddered at the thought of losing it. But with each round, by day 12 or so the sensation was almost gone and I would push back the fear that it would be permanent.

The eighth and final Taxol treatment was rapidly approaching.

FIFTEEN

Taking on the myths of cancer

I was in the midst of those precious good days, and went out for lunch with a friend to celebrate his birthday. He worked at the CBC and seeing him reminded me that I had been meaning to call Wendy Mesley, the CBC journalist who was diagnosed with breast cancer at the same time that I was. I wanted to see how she was doing.

In the course of our conversation she mentioned that an infuriating press release had come across her desk and that both she and I were mentioned in it. The release was put out by the head of a stress-management company. It said, in part:

Given that stress levels and pressures will continue to grow, the strain of the work/life demands upon the modern woman will assuredly mount as well. The high profile cases of cancer afflicting young, famous women like Wendy Mesley, Marla Shapiro, Beverly Thomson . . . only highlights the problem of working professional women strained to the point of dis-ease.

As I got to the paragraph that mentioned my name, I was livid. How dare this person use my name in this way? Not only was the information considered wrong by many medical experts, I felt it was using scare tactics. To suggest that getting breast cancer is the patient's fault and a result of being stressed ("strained to the point of dis-ease") had me in a fury.

My initial reaction was to take this personally and rant and rave. Then I realized that this was just one more opportunity to correct a cancer myth and to reassure women and men that stress does not give you cancer. I decided to write about it, once I had calmed down, and do what I could to debunk this common myth. To that end, I addressed the topic in my *Globe and Mail* column. I did not mention the author's name, since that was not the point. The *Globe* was a platform to educate, and I would not abuse that privilege, as angry as I was. I asked both Wendy Mesley and Bev Thomson if I could reprint the press release and use their names in the article. They were gracious and said yes, anything to correct this manipulation. The column went to press a few months later.

Shelve the blame game: Stress doesn't cause breast cancer

At my most recent appointment with my surgical oncologist at Princess Margaret Hospital, the nurse educator came up to me. She told me that my name came up all the time in her class. Women, diagnosed with breast cancer and wondering what they had done to get this disease, pointed out that I had breast cancer. They would go on to say that certainly

I, as a doctor, must know what to do to prevent breast cancer, and if I could get it, then anyone could. They found it comforting, she said, to know that "even Dr. Marla got breast cancer."

As a practising physician, I am only too aware of the anguish this diagnosis causes, and the self-blame, usually undeserved, that so many women feel. I was particularly infuriated when a release from a stress-management company . . . came across my desk. It argued that "the high profile cases of cancer afflicting young, famous women like [CBC journalist] Wendy Mesley, Marla Shapiro [CTV broadcaster], Beverly Thomson [CTV *Canada AM*] . . . highlights the problem of working professional women strained to the point of dis-ease."

How presumptuous—and how untrue. Not only did it assume that I am "strained to the point of dis-ease" and infer that it was in some way related to the cause of my cancer, but the statement lacks any scientific merit.

As the Canadian Cancer Society points out, there is no single cause of breast cancer but there are factors that increase the risk of developing it. Stress does not appear anywhere on that list.

What are the risk factors for breast cancer? Age is one; while breast cancer can and does appear in women of any age, the risk increases with age.

A family history of breast cancer, especially in a mother, sister or daughter (or if the BRCA1 or BRCA2 gene is present), increases risk. As well, a family history of uterine, colorectal or ovarian cancers increases risk.

If a woman has had previous breast disorders where a biopsy has shown abnormal cells, that too increases risk. Never having been pregnant, a first pregnancy after 30, menstruating at an early age, and later than average menopause are all noted risk factors, as is dense breast tissue and hormone replacement therapy.

As far as diet, obesity and exercise is concerned, several studies are under way probing those possible links. Drinking large amounts of alcohol regularly is linked to a slight increase in breast cancer. Then there are specific risks, such as having radiation therapy to the chest before age 30 (as in therapy used in Hodgkin's disease).

A 2001 study in the International Journal of Cancer, titled "Stress of Daily Activities and Risk of Breast Cancer," notes the belief that life stress enhances breast cancer is common. That study investigated the association between stress of daily activities and breast-cancer risk, and found no evidence of an association between daily stress and breast-cancer risk.

What about stress and recurrence of breast cancer, after diagnosis and treatment? A 2003 study in the British Medical Journal found there was no data to confirm that stressful life experiences increase the risk of recurrence of breast cancer. Its conclusions state that "women with breast cancer need not fear that stressful life experiences will precipitate the return of their disease."

To further probe the relationship between stress and cancer, I queried Dr. Robert Buckman, professor of oncology at Princess Margaret Hospital. "There is no credible evidence whatever that stress itself [as opposed to a behaviour such as smoking cigarettes] contributes to the cause of any cancers, or even affects the course of a cancer," he replied.

"It's easy to see why so many people would like it to be true—because then the patients could be seen as partly 'bringing it on themselves'—but there are many studies showing no connection whatever between stress, bereavement, depression and attitudes with the chance of getting a cancer . . . It has never been, and it is not now, a contributory factor in the causes of cancer."

Stress is known to increase the risk of exacerbating many existing illnesses. But it is without scientific merit, and certainly misleading, to suggest that "working professional women" are "strained to the point of dis-ease." It is clear that many women who develop breast cancer do not have any of the known risk factors.

That is why we cannot explain to such women why they have the disease.

No matter what your lifestyle, or what stresses you face, the best way to help prevent illness of

any sort is to eat well, exercise regularly, keep
your weight in an appropriate range, not drink
to excess, not smoke, accept the support of
friends and family, and enjoy life.

And so, having written the piece, I still did not know what
had caused my cancer. I was still damn angry I had breast
cancer. You can only do your best and move forward, but I
knew that I was not strained in my life. I had made choices, my
choices. Even if at times life was stressful, it sure as hell did not
give me cancer. But I had cancer, and I had made a choice to
fight it. With that in mind I went on to chemotherapy treatment number eight, what I hoped would be the final round.
The gloves went back on.

SIXTEEN

It's no fun having me as a patient

So here I was at the eighth and final chemo. By now I had lost all my eyebrows and my lashes; I was completely hairless. My eyes were constantly tearing from excessive dryness. It was impossible to put on any makeup. My brother-in-law Alan, an ophthalmologist, suggested I use liquid tears in gel form, which was somewhat helpful. Because I had no nasal hairs, my nose would leak large drops of fluid without any warning at all, which I found distressing and embarrassing. It was awful. I felt humiliated by my body.

My friend Susan, who had been there with me for my first chemo, thought it fitting that she take me to the last. I did my usual *Canada AM,* came home and changed and we went off to the hospital. Bobby surprised me and met us there. He wanted to be there for the last one too. Somehow, although I knew this gesture should be met with appreciation, I was neutral. I thanked him, but unlike Bobby and all my friends who were joyful at this final round of treatment, I was numb.

I climbed into my usual bed, got the chemo, promptly fell asleep and awoke to find it over. I had an appointment with

Dr. Trudeau to discuss where we went from there, but she had gone away and I was given her replacement. I was still under sedation, but angry. I wanted Dr. Trudeau. The doctor and I talked about my options for treatment and made a tentative decision for me to start on shots of Zoladex (a drug known generically as goserelin acetate; it is used to stop the production of estrogen) to ensure I was in menopause, and then start anastrozole, which goes by the brand name Arimidex, one of a class of drugs known as aromatase inhibitors.

I went home, unhappy. I felt empty and wondered if it was because I was fearful now that the chemo was over. I had done as much as I could in the way of chemotherapy. What if it didn't work?

I opened my e-mails to see messages from friends congratulating me on finishing the chemo. I fired off nasty responses saying that I had lots more to do and this was no big deal. I don't think I wanted to admit that this part was over. For the past four months my life had revolved around coping with chemotherapy. Despite the work I had been doing, I hadn't allowed myself to think about much else. I don't think I was ready to let go of this place of relative safety and certainty.

I sent off an angry, insecure e-mail to Dr. Trudeau telling her that I understood how busy her schedule was but that I needed to see her and discuss where we would go from here. In her calm and tolerant manner, she replied that she understood that I wanted to see her and perhaps it would have been best to have cancelled the appointment immediately following chemo and waited until she could see me. She had accepted an interim director position, and though I was sincerely proud of and thrilled for her, I also needed to see her. She was my doctor; she had agreed to treat me. We scheduled an appointment for the following week. I was grateful—and apologetic. I wanted to be a good patient, but I was an anxious patient.

And then something exploded. It was my friends. First, I got an angry e-mail from a girlfriend who tersely and briefly wrote in caps—akin to yelling, in an e-mail—that she was "pissed off" with me, that when I wanted to be her friend again I could call, that she was furious I had not answered any of her phone calls. She herself had had breast cancer. I sent off a terse reply telling her that this was about me and if being my friend meant letting me cope in my own way, then so be it. She, having endured chemo, should have known what it was about. I was furious.

Shortly afterwards, a close friend called and told me she needed to see me. She came over and sat down. She started to cry and told me how hard this was for her to say, but she felt that I had excluded her, and her alone. No matter what she said or had written to me, I had snapped back, terse and angry. She didn't know what she had done, and she was terribly hurt. I listened carefully and then I began to talk, slowly and quietly and not quite sure what I was going to say or how I really felt. I told her—but really, when I think about it, I was telling myself—how angry I was, angry to have cancer, angry to put my children through this. I said that I clearly wanted to hang on to the anger and that it was my anger at what was happening—not at her—that was making its way into my e-mails, my refusal to take calls or return messages. I went on, the words now falling out in a rush, about how difficult all of this was, how angry I was that I couldn't imagine getting past it. That there was no reassurance for me. That I knew too much, saw too much, and I wondered if I would ever stop thinking about it coming back, about dying; would I ever live life without feeling this beside me. And that no matter how uncertain all of our lives were, this somehow made me different from the rest of my group of friends. I was the one with cancer. I was the one with no hair. I was the one with a nine-year-old son who now knew what the word *survival* was. I was the one with children who were fearful about their mother dying. I was angry at all of it.

It wasn't until that moment that I realized how angry I actually was and how good a job I had done of putting on my cope-with-it face, my this-isn't-going-to-change-me face, my I-can-do-it-alone face. The words poured out of me and it was a relief. I realized how tough I had been on my friends. She reminded me that she had been tested and I had been tested and I had to stop and realize the overwhelming support I had and how truly lucky I was. And I, more than anyone, knew that. I had to uncover the anger, release it, before I had any hope of getting past it.

That night I sat down and sent a letter to my closest friends, a letter that included the following paragraphs:

So yes indeed it is a milestone of sorts as has been pointed out to me many times this week. The eighth and final chemotherapy of this series has come and gone. So to all of you who have tried to support me despite my difficulty at being supportable, my resistance to taking calls, returning calls and the like, I appreciate all your efforts at putting up with me.

The truth is that there is no right or wrong thing to do. Know that when I appear angry or just unwilling to accept help, it has more to do with me and my anger at being in this position altogether. The truth is that I have no words of wisdom that would help me support anyone else. This is something to endure, and then hopefully let it find its place in my life so it isn't with me every waking moment but more in the background.

Being a doctor is a curse. While it might make me more informed to make decisions, it is clear that I see the dark side of everything. So it is hard to be reassured at the best of times . . . so thank you all, there is still a long way to go. Thanks for being on the ride.

I closed down the computer and sat there for a while. This *was* a milestone. As angry as I was, I had gone through eight rounds of chemotherapy, had had no major adverse events, no hospitalizations, no major infections; my low white-cell counts had been well managed by my shots. I reminded myself to take a breath. I didn't have to be Pollyana. I was allowed to be angry and I was allowed to share it—with my friends, but, more important, with myself.

And then it became very clear. I had wanted to do a documentary on my experience and had accumulated some footage. Not too many people actually film this kind of process, but I had. I began to realize that this was not a documentary about scientific advances, but about life, my family and friends, me, my patients, how this changes the person who experiences it. How it turns you inside out. I felt like I was running every minute of every day, running a race—my race. I could make the choice not to run it alone. My friends insisted that I accept their help and I was getting better at opening up and accepting help. I would tell my story.

My final week of giving myself home injections was also upon me. My thighs were black and blue and sore from the injections and, frankly, each shot hurt a lot. I'd had enough. Matthew was excited and counted off each day, and I was actually getting excited too. Matt's questions showed me that he still had serious matters on his mind.

"Mummy," he said, "if you have cancer, and you don't have the surgery, and you don't take the chemo, and you don't take the needles and you don't go bald, what happens?" I answered quietly that not right away, but with time, with my cancer, you would die. "But Mummy, if you have the surgery, take the chemo, all those needles and go bald, what happens?" I thought long and carefully, realizing that Matt was in fact asking out loud what I had silently asked myself. I told him, softly, slowly, that there were no guarantees about anything in life, but that I had not gone bald for nothing, and that my plans were to be around for a very long time, to yell at him to do his homework, clean his room, brush his teeth, take a shower . . . He started to laugh. I told him, "I will be okay." And I thought, *I have to be okay. I need to be okay.*

The day of my last needle, Matt made a big sign. He goes to French school and his English spelling is a little rough. I had to laugh when a large sign appeared on the fridge that said: TODAY IS YOUR LAST NIDIL. No matter how you spelled it, the fact of my last needle was delightful, thrilling. It felt good and I stopped to enjoy the moment.

The following day I was scheduled to have the portacath removed. Off to Sunnybrook I went and met Dr. Pugash, who greeted me by saying, "That was fast." I laughed and she acknowledged that maybe it hadn't seemed fast for me. But I was indeed there, ready for the port to come out. Dr. Pugash made a tiny incision and worked hard to get me a good cosmetic result. I reminded her that if she left an ugly scar I would tell everyone she had done it, so she'd better do a good job. She smiled tolerantly at me, knowing that I wanted the evidence of my portacath to disappear the same way I hoped the cancer had. She slowly snipped the sutures and dissected the tissue that had grown attached to the port, and suddenly it was out. She washed it off and gave it to me in a sterile urine sample container. I thanked her and headed home, feeling liberated.

Over the next few days I had doctors lined up everywhere.

First, I saw Maureen. She spent a lot of time with me reviewing where we stood and what would happen next. We agreed that one month after the last day of Taxol, I would get an intra-abdominal shot of Zoladex, and another one each month until the hysterectomy, which would ensure by surgical removal of the ovaries that I was in menopause. We also debated the use of Arimidex, the newer aromatose inhibitor drug.

Unlike tamoxifen, until then the gold standard for blocking estrogen receptors in the breast tissue, Arimidex worked at the level of an enzyme to stop "precursor hormones" from making estrogen. A landmark study called the ATAC study had shown improvement in recurrent disease and distant disease compared to tamoxifen. It was being called the new gold standard. There was no survival data yet since this drug had not been around long enough. But it seemed to make sense that if disease-free results were better with Arimidex than with tamoxifen, then survival ultimately would be better as well. Again I was faced with uncertainty about a decision to make. I knew that Dr. Love thought I should have tamoxifen. We chose the aromatase inhibitor Arimidex. The decision was made.

Two days later I went to see Dr. McCready, my breast surgeon. The date of my bilateral mastectomy was approaching. The schedule I had begged for allowed no time for me to take

a breath and recover from the 16 weeks of gruelling chemotherapy. I would not allow myself to admit how ill I really was.
I had unrealistic expectations of myself, but I always have. As
long as my marrow had recovered fully and my counts were
normal, the plan was to have the mastectomies four weeks after
the chemo ended. Then, eight weeks after that, I was booking
the hysterectomy. Two weeks later I was planning to be back
on the road to the Atlantic provinces for a speaking tour on
osteoporosis. Thinking there might be an end to all this, and a
return to the old, familiar me, seemed reassuring. I wondered
if there really was an old, familiar me but pushed that thought
far from my mind.

Dr. McCready and I talked about the surgery and what to
expect. He asked if Maureen had put me on tamoxifen. I told
him we had decided on anastrozole (Arimidex) and he said okay,
but it made me anxious and nervous. He had assumed I would
be on tamoxifen. I began to worry that I had pushed Maureen
in the direction of Arimidex. I knew she would never agree to
do something she did not feel comfortable with, but I couldn't
let go of the thought that somehow I had pushed and that, in
the face of two equivalent treatments, maybe she wouldn't have
suggested this option.

My anxiety increased and I was angry with myself. I
reminded myself she was an expert and could not be swayed
to prescribe a treatment she did not believe in. But I couldn't
let go. I wasn't sure what to do. How could I call yet again
and have this discussion without being insulting or pompous
or just plain irritating? I realized that I was doing exactly what
I told my patients to avoid doing. I was accepting a lot of free
and unsolicited advice, and it was upsetting me. I have always
told my patients that there will always be conflicting opinions,

and therefore to find the source they trust in. In the face of uncertain knowledge, go with the opinion of the doctor you have chosen, not the opinions of those you have not chosen. I was furious with myself, but I couldn't calm down. I had driven the bus—or at least it felt like I had driven the bus—and I had only a learner's permit. Maureen was the bus driver.

I agonized for hours about what to do. In our last visit I had apologized for being difficult and acknowledged how hard it must be to have a patient like me. She told me I was a challenge and that she enjoyed the challenge. I knew she certainly was never intimidated by me, that she understood me and my difficulties in being a patient no matter how hard I tried to be a good patient. But somehow this felt different. Would I be insinuating that she had not been the real decision-maker for my treatment plan? Would I be giving her the message that I didn't believe in her? But it was exactly the opposite. What I had realized was that I didn't believe in myself. I was not, am not an oncologist. And while I am a good doctor, what makes me a better doctor is knowing my own limitations and restrictions.

I decided at last to contact her via e-mail, thinking it would be the least intrusive form of communication. Even so, I thought she might fire me as a patient; I thought she just might have had enough. I sat down and slowly constructed the e-mail. I sent it off.

Dear Maureen,

So I have to start this by fully acknowledging how difficult it must be to be my doctor. How a modicum of knowledge on behalf of the patient must be trying from your point of view. . . . not always, but certainly at times!! And I thank you for indulging my questions.

But now I am anxious that perhaps I have pushed too hard in terms of my opinions and viewpoints. Whatever I do know, I know that I certainly am not an oncologist and more importantly lack your years of expertise, that accumulated experience that accounts for so much of what makes an expert an expert.

What is so difficult about also being me is that I get so much unsolicited advice from physicians . . . the so-called benefit of their experience and free advice. I remind myself and you that I chose you as my oncologist because of my firm respect for your expertise, training and academic knowledge. Above all else you are empathic and patient with me. I know— from my husband as well as the mirror—that that is not always easy.

I saw David McCready for my pre-op. He assumed I would go on tamoxifen first then an aromatase inhibitor. Not an unreasonable expectation. And I won't bother you with the other experts who have added their two cents' worth.

I wanted to settle in my own mind that the decision to put me on Arimidex is one you feel is the best choice for me. I worry that I pushed for this. It is all so confusing—the data on tamoxifen for two years followed by an aromatase inhibitor, the newer ATAC study. . . . More than any other patient I understand the uncertainty of treatment and making decisions based on the best knowledge we have at the moment, and accumulated expertise.

So I wanted to make sure that you are entirely comfortable with the decision to use Arimidex rather than tamoxifen first. I wanted to make sure that you think the TAHBSO [total hysterectomy] is the right thing to do as well.

I cannot imagine for a minute that you could be persuaded to use a treatment plan that you did not feel was equivalent, but I worry that my opinion, voiced as it was, might have swayed you away from what you would have suggested had I not stepped into the fray!! Perhaps you would have suggested tamoxifen.

My initial problem with Dr. Q was that her approach was so equivocal . . . I could do either, and I guess when I pushed the ATAC study, she agreed to Arimidex. I am worried that this then set our discussion in motion on the basis of an opinion that suggested the patient (meaning me) felt strongly about Arimidex.

I am *not* really entitled to feel strongly about *any* treatment option given that indeed I am not an oncologist. You are and it is in you I have put my faith and trust in the direction you point me.

I am trying to cut off these unsolicited opinions. It is the advice I would give my own patients. I should listen to myself with respect to that valuable advice. I must avoid discussion with other prominent cancer patients treated in the same institution who are on different courses with similar tumour types.

So again I apologize entirely for being difficult, anxious and sending you countless e-mails.

I guess I needed to have the conversation one more time about the difference between tamoxifen, then an aromatase inhibitor, versus aromatase inhibitor right from the start.

It is not that I am uncomfortable. I guess I needed to be clear with myself and then with you and apologize for trying to drive the bus!

My bone density today is stable in the hip but down in the back through the entire spine to moderate to severe osteopenia. It appears to be a significant loss but I have asked them to send you the 2003 and today's copy.

Again, thank you for caring for me and putting up with me. I'm getting better at being a patient—or at least I will try!!

My deepest respect,
Marla

That night I went to sleep feeling unhappy and uncomfortable. I knew Maureen was out of town for a week. I would have to sit and wait. And if the e-mail seems really technical, all it really boils down to is yet another agonizing choice under conditions of uncertainty. It is so damn hard to have cancer when there are no clear answers.

I was fortunate that Dr. Trudeau could see what was going on in my head and the anxiety I faced about knowing a lot about a little and realizing that perhaps I had intervened too much. Her response, once she got home to read the e-mail, was swift and reassuring: "You're not a pain in the ass!"

She then went on to review the science of the decision and her opinion that the decision to go directly to Arimidex, rather than tamoxifen, was an entirely reasonable one. But more important, she ended the e-mail with the following:

So, no, you didn't push the discussion in a direction I wasn't already considering. But having said all this, you and I both know there can be more than one right answer. Often we only know what was best in retrospect. Maureen

That was all I really needed to hear. I knew all too well the uncertainty in disease management and could accept the intrinsic uncertainty. What I could not accept was being my own doctor. I had learned a valuable lesson. My oncologist was the expert. I was not. You see, being a doctor does not necessarily mean you know everything in every specialty. While it is important to be informed, in the end it is more important to have a team you trust and can collaborate with. I now had the answer to the question that had been asked of me so many months earlier. It is important to have the doctor whom you believe knows the most about you and the science, and to let him or her guide you through this maze.

PART THREE

THE VIEW FROM HERE

SEVENTEEN

The next chapter

The chemo was over. But without that familiar pattern and routine, I was uncomfortable and worried. With chemo, I knew what to expect. Now I wasn't entirely sure how to navigate what was ahead. But more and more I felt the need to tell my story.

Out of the blue I heard from Vicki Gabereau, who had a daytime talk show in Vancouver. Late the previous summer I had been asked to appear on the show to promote *Balance*. I had declined, claiming a busy schedule, but that was before it was general knowledge that I had breast cancer. Now, frustrated that my own network had not moved on or returned any e-mails concerning a network special, I asked Vicki to invite me on her show again. Her answer was immediate; she scheduled me for a segment. We arranged for me to fly down at once, since my timing was limited: I had only four weeks between chemo ending and the upcoming mastectomies. I thought long and hard and decided I wanted the focus to be on my breast cancer. I did have a message to share. I also decided I would be me, which meant, among other things, going bald.

I had not been wearing the wig anywhere in my real life and would not do so on Vicki's show either. Bald in real life is one thing; bald on national television is another. But it felt wrong to wear it and I did not want to bring it and talk myself into wearing it. The wig was not me. The bald woman looking back from the mirror was me. I was comfortable with her, the evolving me, and I realized that was all that counted. So, 18 days after my last chemo, I boarded a plane, bald and wigless, and flew to Vancouver. I did not ask permission from my oncologist. I knew my white-cell counts were still low but I didn't care. I knew a plane was a risky environment for catching illnesses but I didn't care. I just did not care.

As I sat on the set with Vicki it became clear there was a lot to talk about. We ended up doing 30 minutes, the entire show. I told Vicki to consider herself uncensored; she could ask any question at all. I talked about what this had been like, how difficult it was, why I was wigless and why I chose to wear a wig on *Canada AM*. The truth, of course, was that I wore a wig so that *Balance* viewers would not see a bald Dr. Marla on *Canada AM* and the "before" Dr. Marla on *Balance*. The latter shows had been pre-taped before I lost my hair. I also said that I didn't want the viewer distracted by my baldness when I was appearing as an expert. We talked about courage and bravery but the truth, I felt, was that I had neither.

This look had chosen me, I told Vicki, but I had decided to embrace it as part of who I had become. Vicki is a tough interviewer. She asked me what was next. I was not prepared to speak publicly yet about the mastectomies, not wanting to discuss them until they were done. I answered that I was weighing my options between radiation and surgery, though in fact all my friends and family knew about my decision and the surgical date of February 15 had been set for some time. I shifted the conversation to my family, my friends, how this had changed me and what a difficult road this was, not only physically gruelling but also emotionally devastating.

The response to the show—the e-mails, the calls, the outcry, the thanks—was overwhelming. I did not expect it. The network did not expect it. Finally my own network sat up and took notice. While I had been asking since November to film what was happening to me—the treatment, the hair loss and so on—they had failed to respond. Admittedly I was angry. Prior to my appearance on *The Vicki Gabereau Show*, my former producer at CityTV contacted me to ask if they could do a special. I told CTV about it but the only response I got was that it would not be looked on favourably. My anger grew. I could not understand why other networks were interested in interviewing me but my own network was ignoring me, often not answering my e-mails. As a medical journalist I knew and understood that decisions at media outlets are often made slowly. But I was angry at having cancer, and that anger was often hard to face. It was much easier to displace that anger, to put it somewhere. The network, in fact, was concerned about me, concerned about putting out such a personal story, which is what I had promised it would be—I could not see the point of telling the story if it was edited and censored. They were being protective of me, but I imagined them wondering too if the show would be watched.

I bumped into the network president in makeup one morning and asked her if we could meet. It was 10 days prior to my surgery and I needed to make some decisions. I wanted to know if CTV was going to support the making of my documentary. I also had no idea if *Balance* was coming back. I had always jumped through hoops for the network by rescheduling patients to meet taping demands, but I was not prepared to do this now. After being away so many months with no end in sight, with a loyal patient population waiting for me, I wanted to set my schedule and cast it in stone. I felt I deserved an answer and an acknowledgement that indeed I had another career that limited my availability. Angry. Angry. Anger was a quiet enemy that walked with me a lot at that time.

I was told to come in the following Monday following a taping for *Canada AM* and Newsnet. I was busy taping stories for Newsnet to cover the time when I would be away.

The next day I had an appointment with my plastic surgeon, Joan Lipa. She measured me, photographed me and answered all my questions. My girlfriend Susan sat through this with me, listening. Though as a non-physician, she understood everything because Joan was so clear in describing the procedure.

Dr. Lipa would draw incision margins on my breast and Dr. McCready would do the bilateral mastectomy. Then Dr. Lipa would continue, opening the pectoral muscles and the serratus anterior, and inserting expanders between the chest wall and muscles, as well as a temporary fill bag with a magnetic port. She would put as much saline as possible into the fill bag, and then close me. I would come for regular fills of saline until my new breasts (actually "chest mounds," to be technically correct!) reached a size that was appropriate from a surgical perspective and also from the perspective of what I hoped to achieve aesthetically. She would then go back in, remove the expanders and the temporary fill bag and replace them with silicone, which I had chosen. This process would span a minimum of six months.

She meticulously went over complications ranging from severe pain, infection, loss of skin and delayed infection—

nothing was spared. The immediate concern was my intolerance of morphine and related drugs, since we knew that I reacted to these with a histamine release, which causes severe itching. We were not sure how to handle this, but I was booked for a preoperative anesthesia consult. Listening to Joan describe all of this, I was nervous but not anxious, if one can make a distinction between the two.

The consult with anesthesia was the next day, and again I was accompanied by a girlfriend. The anesthesiologist and I reviewed my latex allergy, which would dictate no latex gloves and a completely latex-free operating room. I am not an easy patient. We decided to try a medication called Dilaudid (which is generically called hydromorphone hydrochloride) as a morphine substitute. Everything was in place. I went for blood work and then my friend and I went for lunch (though I could only sip at the wine she insisted we order to celebrate this next phase) and then shopping. Anything to distract.

Late that same afternoon, I got a frantic call from Joan's office. My white-cell count was terrible. The surgery could not go on as planned with such low counts. I stopped dead in my tracks. I could not accept a change in schedule, could not have a delay. I needed to have control of the what and the when. As usual I had planned everything meticulously, and if one surgery got delayed the whole plan would fall apart. I wanted to see the end of the road, the end of the tunnel. I was unrealistic but refused to accept that. I have always refused to accept that about myself.

I was advised to call my oncologist, Dr. Trudeau. I did that immediately but she was not there on a Friday at 4 p.m. Her secretary would try to find her. In the meantime, I had her e-mail address and I knew she had a Blackberry; I sent an urgent message. She called me back and we arranged to meet at the hospital pharmacy so that I could pick up some Neulasta, which is a longer-acting white-cell stimulator than Neupogen. I was stunned that Maureen came to meet me. She could have just phoned in the prescription but I think she wanted to make sure I really could go ahead safely with the surgery; she could hear the panic in my voice. My friend and I raced to the hospital, where Maureen met me. I was so grateful for her dedication. My drug plan refused to cover the medication, so some $2,700 later I went home and injected myself and prayed.

The following Monday morning I went to the CTV boardroom and was shocked to find not only the executive producer of my show, but three other people representing variety programming, network news and *Canada AM*. I had no idea why they were there. The president was not there; I knew she was busy with CTV's joint bid, with Rogers Communications, for the 2010 and 2012 Olympics.

The meeting started with them asking me why I had called it. Though they already knew the agenda, I began to outline my vision for *Balance*, how I would keep it exciting and current, and explained that taping a year's worth of programming in three and a half months was limiting and unrealistic. They let me ramble on, but I wondered why I was doing all the speaking. I stopped—and was told there would be no money for *Balance*, no season three. Despite our hit ratings, we were not being renewed. The head of the production company that produced *Balance* later told me that he had never had a hit show not be renewed, but my friend Valerie Pringle told me that good shows get cancelled all the time: it is simply the way of the television world. Though I accepted the network's decision—I had no choice—I found it remarkable, another huge loss.

Moreover, I was furious about the way in which the message had been delivered. I was not sure why representatives from network news and *Canada AM* were there. I wanted this news to be told to me privately, individually. Of course, *Canada AM* and the network news divisions also employ me, and they were present that day to let me know that this was not a personal decision. My relationship with Newsnet would continue; I would still be the network's medical consultant. The network played it straight, the way it should have been played: here are the facts, now let's move on. Being an angry woman, though, I experienced this as just one more thing to be angry about.

I knew I was not being rational. *Balance* was not my child. My children were at home. *Balance* was a job I loved doing. I had done a good job, and it had been an honour and a fabulous experience. Lack of funds in the television industry is a way of life. This was not personal. This was reality. I took some deep breaths, tried to stay calm. In any case, I reminded myself, the truth was that I had already decided I would not come back to the show if the taping schedule remained the same. Anywhere from eight to ten shows per week, plus my full-time medical practice . . . I was not prepared to work that way again and rob my family of me. I was embarrassed at myself, at how selfishly I had made decisions. Truth be known, I had been selfish about my career, which I had learned the day I watched Amanda's induction as a prefect. I had learned that lesson and now needed to translate it into action. The network had made it easy for me.

The next part of the meeting was the good news: they did indeed want a network special about my story. I knew that we had footage from my appearances on *Canada AM* and *Vicki,* as well as my own footage. We could do this. But when the president finally got a minute to run in, I told her that I felt as if I had been "shown the door." She reassured me, as the others had, that my relationship with network news and *Canada AM* had not changed. It was time to move on with new projects, which included them trusting me and believing in me to write and produce my own network prime-time special. This was an enormous show of faith, an enormous offer of support. And they had given me complete latitude to do this on my own, to tell my story in my own way. The import of that message began to sink in.

Together with CTV, I had branded myself, and "Dr. Marla" was a known entity. Now the network had opened the birdcage door and it was up to me to fly. They believed I could fly, and for that, for the belief they had always had in me, I was enormously grateful.

That night there was an end-of-chemo party for me. My sister-in-law Wendy had sent out invitations with a personalized rewriting of "My Favorite Things" from *The Sound of Music*. It was hilarious. Thankfully I could see the humour and let go of some of the anger left over from the day's meeting.

Ketel One on Ice and chocolate almonds by Hershey
Chapman's Biscotti and vanilla yogurt fat free
Peanut butter and banana sandwiches put her in the mood
These are a few of her favourite foods.
Greek salad and crisp apple strudel
Seared tuna and schnitzel with noodles
Sushi rolls with ginger and noodle puddings
These are a few of Marla's footings.
Baked Lays in bags and Diet Dr. Pepper cans
Fresh fruit, lattes and hot apple flan

Crisp edamame and cappuccino Skor bar
These are a few of Marla's favourites by far.
When the scale sings
When the phone rings
When she's feeling sad
She simply remembers her favourite foods
And then she doesn't feel so bad.
Please join us for an END OF CHEMO PARTY!!!!
HURRAY!!! HURRAY!!!

I had been reluctant about the party. Leading up to it I felt that nothing had really ended, and now with my low white-cell count I feared that the surgery was threatened. But I remembered that the party was being given by all the friends who had supported me. Some wonderful things had already come out of this horrible experience. During my chemotherapy treatments my sister-in-law Sandy had been on sabbatical from teaching and had been a wonderful support; we had established a really important friendship. I had learned about the strength of my friends and how lucky, truly lucky, I was. Yes, with the end of chemo a page had been turned in this story and a large part of the treatment was over. There might even have been a little fuzz returning to my head.

I got dressed and went to the party. Admittedly, it was fun. All my favourite foods were waiting, from peanut-butter-and-banana pinwheel party sandwiches on whole wheat to chocolate almonds and even a cappuccino-Skor Blizzard, my absolute all-time favourite Blizzard. My appetite was still not terrific but I appreciated the love and energy that had gone into the party. My sister and her daughter had flown in to surprise me and I was indeed surprised—*no one* pulls anything over on me, ever, and they had surprised me! I was overwhelmed. She also brought me what I had asked her to send: loot bags, comprising one item, for each of my friends. I got up and told everyone gathered how much they all meant to me, thanked them for their support and told them that if I was getting new ones, so should they . . . With that, I gave each of my girlfriends a chocolate boob-on-a-stick, complete with pink nipple.

Amanda would turn 18 on February 16, the day after my impending surgery. I had taken Jenna away when she turned 18 and wanted to do the same with Amanda. On the darkest days, retrieving memories from such times is a gift. It was Amanda's last year of high school, an important final semester for her, but we knew this time together was precious and so, despite the pressures she felt at school, she took the week off. The next morning, as my sister and niece flew home, Amanda and I flew off together for six days in Florida.

We concentrated on relaxing. We went to the gym, sat at the pool, shopped for a formal dress for her and just enjoyed being together. We both knew what I faced when we went home. Neither of us talked about it.

Everyone had odd stares and comments about my bald head, including a hairdresser who offered to make me a wig if I flew to New York. When I gently told him I *chose* to go around this way, he was amazed. I reassured him and laughed at how my hairlessness made everyone else feel naked! Wigs, I could now conclude with total confidence, were for other people's comfort, not mine.

The night before we went home Amanda developed food poisoning and spent the evening throwing up in the bathroom. As supportive as I tried to be, I couldn't help but laugh: I had escaped chemo vomit-free. We ordered room service and watched television together. I knew I still had a role to play as her mother; my job was not done.

We flew home the next morning, ready to face the upcoming week. At the other end, Bobby was waiting. As supportive as ever, he had allowed me to call the shots throughout this whole ordeal, letting me do what I thought I needed to do. He was glad to see us, to see me. It was the day before Valentine's Day and two days before my surgery. I was ready. I was nervous, but I was ready.

EIGHTEEN

Off with their heads, so to speak

I felt a little like Alice in Wonderland. I wasn't exactly sure how I had gotten to this point.

Breast cancer sets off a cascade of decision-making. Decisions have to be made, and made quickly. No matter how much you think them through, there is always that sense of urgency to make a quick decision and make the right decision. David had been abundantly clear: a bilateral mastectomy was not his choice. Time and time again he pointed out that the risk of recurrence was 10% with or without the mastectomy. With the 10% of cancers that do recur after mastectomy, the recurrence is usually in the suture or incision line. And of course if that happens, the cancerous cells are right beside the muscle wall, with no breast to buffer that recurrence.

But I couldn't escape the thought that we had missed the ductal carcinoma in situ by mammogram and it had been picked up only when it had become invasive. I would never feel confident that there wasn't something lurking in the remaining breast or that something wasn't already lurking in my so-called healthy breast. And while, yes, the 10% recurrence rate would be the same on the right breast, there would be a 90% reduction of risk in my healthy breast. More important, I would not live from test to test holding my breath and wondering if the MRI or mammogram was accurate. Dr. Love told me that my breasts would get fatty over time, and would therefore become easier to examine through mammography. But I had over 90% dense tissue. Dr. Bukhanov felt that the fatty tissue would accumulate very slowly and my breasts would therefore be dense for years to come.

So there I was on the morning of February 15, a deadly calm having descended over me.

Susan and Renee met Bobby and me at the hospital. It was 6 a.m. I was the first case of the day because of my latex allergy. The four of us sat there waiting as the nurses went through the motions of taking my blood pressure, temperature and so on—my "vitals." When I was ready to be moved to the OR bed and await Joan and David, I was told that I could have only two people accompany me. Without hesitating I tossed off, "Bye, Bobby." The girls laughed, Bobby laughed and the nurse relented. We were a team. I had come to accept that this was part of my recovery, accepting their love and support, their distractions.

Both Susan and Renee were surprised that I was so calm. But the decision had been made and I refused to revisit it. I was there. My breasts were coming off. And yes, it had been a difficult decision, not as easy as I thought it would be. As I had realized in discussions with Maureen, I do not identify myself with my breasts, but rather my brain. Offered a lobotomy as a life-saving strategy, I would have said no, taken my chances and probably died prematurely. But I had been examining breasts for years as a physician. They were just another body part, or so

I told myself. Still, I knew my body image was about to change and my body was about to be brutalized. I refused to dwell on that. I would later say in an interview that the night before the surgery I looked at myself in the mirror, looked at my breasts and thought, *You are not my friends.* And with that I could say good night and goodbye.

Joan came to me in the OR bed with a marker to mark the undersides of my breasts for where the normal landmarks are. Once David took the breasts off, she would need a "road map" to place the expanders. I told her to tell David to take more skin along the incision line. My cancer had been very close to the skin margin and I wanted a wider excision. But she reminded me that David would not know where along the incision line the cancer had been and if he widened the removal of skin along all 7 centimetres, the skin would be compromised, and perhaps the cosmetic result as well.

I was about to have what is called a skin-sparing mastectomy. In other words, as much as possible, the breast tissue is scooped out like the inside of a hard-boiled egg. It is impossible to take out 100% of the tissue. David would preserve as much skin as possible so that it could be put back together and stretched over time to accommodate the expanders as they got larger. I did not care. I had come this far and it was not about cosmetics. It was about my family, my life. I did not care.

At my request, Joan used the indelible marker to write over the incision line: "Take more, take more." We laughed to think what David's reaction might be. Joan became quiet as she methodically marked the underside of the breasts, how far they were from the sternum (chest bone), and around the nipples that would soon be gone. I knew when I awoke I would look very different.

We waited for what seemed like an eternity and finally it was time. Renee and Susan kissed me, Bobby kissed me, and I flashed them one last time as I told them to say goodbye to the girls, my affectionate name for my soon-to-be-lost breasts.

I got into the OR and the anesthetist got ready to start the IV and sedate me. David walked in and smiled. Now my surgical team was here. Each was essential: David to painstakingly take as much tissue as he possibly could; Joan to start me on the long and painful road to reconstruction. I was already groggy as David came over to talk to me. I told him I had left him a message, and flashed my chest. Dr. McCready is a caring, wonderful surgeon but I think I was just a little different from most of his other patients. Somewhat surprised, but then again, not entirely—this was me—he read the message and knew that I understood it might compromise the cosmetic results. He reminded me that he felt the margins were adequate, but that yes, confident that I could give him informed consent, he would indeed take more. As I drifted off, I was calm, knowing there was no turning back. None.

I awoke in recovery. As I'd been warned, the pain was excruciating. I felt like two elephants were sitting on my chest, or that a rubber band was being pulled tighter and tighter across my chest. The movement of my chest with my breathing was horrible. I tried to pace myself, to reach deep inside to my own personal pain control. More than anything, I tried not to move. I had drains, two in each breast, connected to four vacuum packs that would help remove the blood and serous fluid that was weeping in my chest and keep the fluids from moving the expanders out of position.

When you have tissue expanders put in during mastectomy, it is unlike inserting expanders for a normal breast augmentation.

With mastectomy, there are no breasts to put the implants under; you have only skin and muscle left. So the muscles of the chest wall had been lifted and the expanders were slid between the chest wall and the ripped muscles. The expanders each had 100 millilitres or so of fluid in them at this point. Muscles are not accepting of aggressive expansion; they're not meant to be. Imagine a hard workout where your muscles are strained. In this case the muscles had been taken off the wall, cut and dissected to house these tissue expanders. The clear, non-latex Opsite dressing on my chest allowed me to see exactly what I looked like. I had learned—painfully—that I cannot tolerate adhesives, so there were no bandages to hide what had been done.

As the nurses prepared to move me I reminded them that no one was to touch me. My close friend and office manager, Barb, had told me that in the excruciating pain after surgery, the worst part for her was when she was moved from the recovery room bed to the hospital bed. To avoid this, I had been doing sit-ups from a lying position for weeks with Stacy, my personal trainer. I was determined to control what I could and no one, *no one*, was going to touch me. When it came time for the bed transfer, with sheer determination I sat up in one full motion, silently thanking Stacy for my toned abdominal muscles. I thought I would pass out from the pain, but it was better than having anyone touch me.

I had been told I would have no use of my arms, that the pain would limit movement altogether. I could not imagine ever brushing my teeth again or wiping myself in the bathroom. I thought it was a good thing I had no hair; that was one thing less to brush.

After a while Joan came by the recovery room and told me that indeed the extra skin removal on the right side had limited how much fluid she could initially put in the expanders. She was confident that with time the muscles would relax and the skin would stretch. In two weeks she would inject more saline through the magnetic port in my expanders. I winced at the thought. She told me to wear a sports bra. That too made me wince. I couldn't imagine getting my arms through anything over my head. In preparation for this I had bought some loose, zip-front sweatshirts. But as prepared as I was, I was unprepared. This really was no fun. Reading about something is not the same as doing it.

Early on Friday morning, a mere two days later, I was begging to be released. When Joan agreed, my sister-in-law Wendy happened to be with me. I did not want to wait for Bobby to get me and so Wendy wheeled me to her sports car. It was a great-looking vehicle, but so low to the ground that every bump translated into agonizing pain. I don't know if the drive home was harder for Wendy or for me. I tried to keep my grimaces to a minimum but she knew I was in agony. Finally we got me in the house, up the nearly insurmountable stairs to my bedroom, and finally, finally into my bed. I was in terrible pain but so very glad to be home. The four vacuum packs draining fluids from my chest wall were pinned to my sweatshirt.

Wendy stayed and Renee came over to be with me as well. I was resting in bed when I suddenly felt wet and sticky. I was hemorrhaging from one of the drains and there was blood everywhere. Bobby wasn't home yet, but Jenna, Wendy and Renee were there. Quietly, my medical training kicked into gear. I told them to get me to the bathroom, get a plastic table-cloth (a Barbie tablecloth from when the girls were little) and place it on the bed (that part was not medical training, but housewife training: I know that blood is hard to remove). I asked for gauze and we applied pressure but I knew I had to get back to the hospital.

Vivien Brown, my family doctor, had been there earlier; Jenna got her on her cell phone and she turned around and came right back. Three of the four drains were working but clearly this one was not, and I was concerned it would compromise the implant. My girlfriends, knowing how awful the drive home had been, were reluctant to move me, but Renee had a van and we felt it would be the best. They packed me up and got me in the van and drove back down to the hospital. We left Jenna at home with Matt. Bobby met us at the hospital. Viv and Bobby came into the ER with me and one of the four drains was removed. The removal of the drain felt like a hot wire being pulled out of my chest. I could have had home care visits in the coming days but we agreed that Vivien would continue to see me at home and remove the remaining three drains as the fluids diminished. I was in pain but anxious to get back home.

Jenna was home, since it was reading week at her university, and it fell to her, during the day, to help me wash, get dressed, go to the bathroom and just move around. But in my usual I-can-do-it way, I took myself to my closet and managed to get a sports bra on through a series of agonizing maneuvers. Then, unable to life my arms, I couldn't get it off. Jenna was ready to kill me. She reminded me to stop rushing it and be a patient. Both of us were in a sweat by the time we got me out of the sports bra and back to bed. (Later, I would think back to my pure stubbornness—what Jenna referred to as stupidity—and wonder that I had not simply cut it off.)

To force myself to relax I reminded myself how terrible the hemorrhage had been, and managed to do very little. I was comforted by the thought that I had written my columns for the *Globe* ahead of time, refusing to take a hiatus; there would be no interruption to that, at least.

Within another few days the fluids draining into the vacuum packs had subsided and the packs were ready to be removed. Each of the three was pulled through the incision that had been left open on the side of the chest wall. The pain, although searing, was brief. At least the round vacuum packs that were pinned to my sweatshirt were gone and I felt a little more human.

That night the Grammys were on, and as I saw Melissa Etheridge bald on the red carpet, I thought, *You go, girl; that is what we look like.* When she got up and sang that primal scream, I felt as if I could scream too. It amazed me how universal were the feelings of women going through this. I did not know then that I would have the opportunity to sit down and do a personal interview with her later that year, almost a year from the date of my first chemotherapy.

For the first two weeks after surgery, I had extremely limited use of my arms. I could not raise them in any way because the muscles were sore and healing. But I could show my chest to anyone who came to visit. Dr. Lipa had created small chest mounds, as she referred to them, with the expanders and the initial expansion. I did look odd. There were no nipples, only two long incisions across the chest wall where my breasts had once been. I did not feel mutilated, as I had been warned that I might. Instead, I marvelled at how amazing this really was.

After two weeks I went back to see Joan. I was entirely numb over my chest wall. She used a magnet to find the magnetized ports under the skin in my chest and then, using a long needle, she injected another 75 millilitres or so into each expander.

Although I could not feel the needle enter I could feel pressure as the fluid was injected. Again, that rubber-band-like sensation returned to my chest wall. Joan assured me the sensation would subside as the fluid distributed itself more evenly in the expanders and the muscles relaxed to accept the expansion.

I was also ready to start the Zoladex injections. Although I had not had a period since the first day of chemo, menopause is defined as the absolute cessation of periods for one year. Given my age, there was a chance that my periods might return. While I waited for the hysterectomy, which was more than a month away, I was given a large injection of Zoladex in my abdominal wall, just under the skin, in a "depot injection." That means the active ingredient—in this case, a luteinizing hormone–releasing analogue (the hormone that ultimately controls ovarian function)—is suspended in a sustained-release vehicle. That vehicle releases slowly, over time, to ensure there is no production of hormone.

Again I was thrust into horrible night sweats and hot flashes. Sleep was a nightmare, disturbed several times each night as I was awakened by the dampness and cold. I would have to warm up, dry off and change the sheets. While I had initially had menopausal symptoms with the first few chemos, that side effect had eventually stopped. Now these symptoms were back with a vengeance.

It was a month after surgery and we were scheduled to go to Palm Desert for March break. I had a speaking engagement and felt well enough to do it. Joan provided me with a letter for airport security that explained I had magnetized ports and would set off the metal detectors. She reminded both Bobby and me that I was not to carry anything. I was allowed to lift light objects, though, since the range of motion in my arms was now near normal; Joan had started me on several gentle stretching exercises at home.

Sitting on the plane I suddenly began to experience excruciating pain in the midsection of my right upper arm. It was intolerable. By the time we landed I felt terrible. The arm looked normal. There was no swelling or redness but the pain literally took my breath away. I lived on painkillers for the week, waiting to go home and see what had happened.

Upon my return I had an ultrasound and x-ray. I knew it was unlikely that I had cancer in my bones at this early stage, but all cancer patients, I imagined, lived with such thoughts for the rest of their lives. Every unexplained anything must be cancer. While I knew as a physician that was not the case, emotionally I could not leave that thought alone.

The ultrasound revealed that the pectoral muscle had torn in the place where it is anchored to the arm. This was entirely understandable. Joan told me that my right chest wall muscles were more difficult to dissect away from the chest. Somewhere during recovery I must have lifted or moved the wrong way and completed a partial tear in the muscle, which might have been there from the surgery or from years of weight-bearing activity. I started ultrasound therapy, massage and physiotherapy, and gradually the pain began to lessen.

I had visits with Joan every few weeks to add more fluid to the expanders. As the skin was scant on the right side we often were limited as to the amount of fluid that could go in at any one time. But gradually the expanders began to fill out—and my chest wall began to look really odd. The expanders are designed so that only the lower two-thirds expand. The top of the expander does not, since those muscles are meant to stay adherent to the chest wall. When the final exchange is done and an implant is put in, the implant will not ride up the chest; instead, it stays put.

I began to look square. As the top of the expander does not enlarge, I had what looked like a shelf. I jokingly called it my martini shelf, as I felt like I could balance a glass on it. I was unable to drink a martini, but I could indeed balance a glass. My family began calling me Sponge Bob Square Boobs, after a cartoon character my son often watched on television.

Things were moving along quickly. The hysterectomy was looming large; it would soon be upon me.

NINETEEN

My other Joan

Dr. Joan Murphy was going to perform the hysterectomy. We met to discuss the procedure and she mentioned that there was a criticism to be made about removing healthy organs. My actual risk for ovarian cancer was pretty small. We had established that I was gene-negative, meaning I did not have the BRCA 1 or 2 mutations. The baseline risk for ovarian cancer might be quoted at around 2%. Having had breast cancer doubled that risk, even in gene-negative women, but that still only put me at 4%.

Another fact to consider on the plus side was that once my ovaries were removed I would be in surgical menopause, without any chance whatever of my periods returning, and I could then take the aromatase inhibitor without any hesitation. The aromatase inhibitor was indicated for use in postmenopausal women only, and while the Zoladex had put me into menopause for the time being, a hysterectomy would seal the deal, so to speak. We spoke about the risks and complications. I had had four previous Caesarean sections, which meant that it would be difficult to perform the hysterectomy through a laparoscopic incision (two small incisions on the abdomen and one on the belly button). The previous surgeries had left a lot of scar tissue, and adhesions would likely have developed over time. I was aware that the surgery might be difficult and Dr. Murphy might have to revert to an open incision, the more traditional way of performing hysterectomy. I was not keen on the idea of the open incision: the greater risks and the longer recovery period after the operation. Still, I wanted to be as aggressive as I could, within reason. I felt that the surgical menopause would not only allow me to take the Arimidex but also let me forget about any possible ovarian or uterine disease. And so, feeling I was closing one more door that needed closing, I agreed to the hysterectomy, and in the middle of April returned yet again for a 6 a.m. surgical call with Bobby and Renee and Susan by my side.

I was in the operating room a long time. My support team told me later they had begun to get anxious. My sister had flown in that morning (my breast cancer was curing her fear of flying) and was with them, pacing. I had discouraged my parents from coming in. My two sisters-in-law and mother-in-law were there too, but I did not surface in the recovery room until the end of the day. As I'd been warned, the surgery had been difficult—even slightly more difficult than had been anticipated. While operating, there had been some difficulty dissecting the uterus from the bladder (the uterus sits in very close proximity to the bladder). There had also been a lot of bleeding, which apparently had been difficult to control. But Joan had managed to complete the surgery through the tiny keyhole incisions.

When I did awake at the very end of the day I had terrible pain and massive swelling on the upper left side of my neck.

None of the nurses had any idea what had happened to me and there was no note in the chart. It was infuriating to me, since I knew I was not crazy. It looked like I had been bitten by a vampire—which, in a sense, as it turned out, I had. The anesthetist finally showed up after being paged several times, and related that during the surgery, when I began losing blood, she had tried to get to a vein to see how low my counts had dropped. Apparently she had some difficulty and chose to draw a blood sample from my neck vein. It was clear she had had some more difficulty and I had bled around her puncture, developing a large amount of swelling and bruising. Joan had been busy operating at her end and had had no idea what was going on up at my neck. No dressing or pressure pack or ice had been applied and the area got more and more tender while I was in recovery. I was furious at the lack of communication. The nurses brought an ice pack to apply to my neck.

Joan arrived and reviewed what had happened—the technical difficulties, the bleeding. And now there were new concerns: with the dissection of the uterus from the bladder wall, she thought the bladder might have been compromised. *Compromised*: it's a word we use often in medicine. The bladder wall looked thin, she said, and she would be sending me home with a catheter in place to drain the bladder for at least a week. She did not want the bladder expanding. She made arrangements for me to meet with a urologist. I was horrified. Although I'd been aware of all these possible complications at the time of signing the consent, they were now a reality. I was fearful that a truly elective procedure would now cause me unwanted complications that I would have to cope with forever. The thought of loss of bladder function plummeted me into a deep state of anxiety. I could see myself walking around with a catheter and urine bag for the rest of my life.

I went home within 24 hours, wanting to escape the hospital. Matt wanted to know why I had a bag of apple juice by my bedside. I did not want to tell him it was urine—he had seen and heard way too much already. My blood counts had dropped precipitously and I was weak. My sister stayed with me that week, intercepting calls and visitors. I didn't want to see anyone at all.

One week later Bobby and I were to go back to the hospital. The night before I spiked a temperature and was afraid that I had developed a urinary tract infection. That would not have been unusual, given that I was living with a bag hanging out of me. I spoke with Joan; she started some antibiotics and told me to get an ultrasound of my bladder and pelvis before my appointment with the urologist.

The ultrasound showed a large mass in the left lower pelvis. The radiologist was afraid it was an abscess. But in spite of a lot of left lower quadrant pain, I felt pretty well otherwise and could not believe a mass the size of a cantaloupe could be an abscess without my being more ill. Joan and I both thought it was a collection of blood that had organized itself into a large bruise (a hematoma, in medical language), and we chose to let it get better on its own and follow up with ultrasound.

I went off to see the urologist, Dr. John Trachtenberg, who performed a cystoscopy. This meant using a small scope equipped with a camera and a light to examine the interior of my bladder. He felt the bladder was healthy and the catheter could come out. My bladder was irritated—just like me—and had only a small capacity before it would go into spasm. Simply put, I felt like I had to urinate all the time. He assured me this was temporary and my bladder capacity would return to normal. I felt I was almost out of the woods except for this undiagnosed collection in my pelvis. I kept reminding myself that this was elective surgery and I had agreed to the risk of these complications.

I went back for serial ultrasounds and the radiologist felt the mass was getting larger. She wanted to put a needle in and attempt to drain it. But I felt well, looked better and had no real signs that this was worrisome. I had no fever. The pain was almost gone and my appetite was better. Both Joan and I agreed that watching and waiting was the best course. I decided I would have no more ultrasounds until or unless I began to feel worse. I knew (or at least hoped) that my body would tell me if I was getting worse. Months later I went back for an ultrasound that showed no further sign of the unidentified mass; this was proof that it had been a collection of blood that had resolved itself.

The hot flashes and night sweats started all over again. This must be it, I thought, the end of the road; it couldn't get any worse. The days weren't bad but the nights were wicked. I was perpetually sleep-deprived. Fortunately, over the next month the symptoms slowly began to abate. If I watched my diet and— for whatever reason—avoided chocolate, the night sweats were manageable. Exercise was key for me and helped minimize the symptoms.

I had had enough. I didn't want to be a patient anymore. Bobby reassured me that there was an end in sight. We were almost done with the surgeries. My birthday was approaching and both Joans gave us clearance to go away. We decided that a few days away with friends, in some warm place, would be just what the doctor needed.

We made our plans and I packed, but I did not have a suitable bathing suit. Any woman will tell you that buying a bathing suit is her least favourite type of shopping. Try it with square expanders for breasts. Anything with an underwire would press against the expanders and cause a lot of discomfort. Anything with a moulded cup would allow a glimpse of my oddly shaped martini-shelf implants. I needed some help. Off I went to a store that specializes in lingerie and bathing-suit fitting.

This particular store has a section that caters to women who have had mastectomies. With my large, squarish, partially filled expanders, however, I was a new challenge for them. I was odd looking. I asked the saleswoman to come in and look at what I was talking about, as it might help her figure out what I could possibly wear. Reluctantly she took a peek. We tried on dozens of styles, looking for anything that would be comfortable and not make me look as unusual as I actually did. I was just about to give up and decide to wear T-shirts over a bikini bottom when the saleswoman found a high-necked bathing suit with a liner but no real cups. We had a small mountain of bathing suits on the floor that had all been rejected: underwires, moulded cups that were way too optimistic for my chest, low-cut halters that stood away from my chest and gave an unwelcome view, bandeau tops that accentuated the squareness of my implants . . . I laughed at how this looked. While I did not have a distorted body image (as I had been warned might be the case), I realized how crazy I had become that this was normal for me. I had accepted how my body looked for the moment, but it *was* unusual.

I was ready for a holiday. I just wished I could have left the new—and somewhat odd-looking—me at home. I was pushing hard to move forward and be normal. But the truth was, it was not easy. Not at all.

TWENTY

Barbie is not anatomically correct

I had been warned about "dysmorphic body syndrome." The medical definition describes a person with this syndrome as being "obsessively preoccupied" with a particular body part that he or she considers unattractive. The syndrome can range from mild to severe. Excessive concern about a "physical anomaly" becomes a preoccupation, and distresses the person enough to interfere with work and social or interpersonal functioning.

I did not have dysmorphic body syndrome, but as time went on, I felt odd. The reconstructive surgery had been entirely successful. Dr. Lipa had done a great job and all that was left was the final "exchange" surgery in July. At that time the temporary (now square) expanders would be removed and replaced with the permanent implants. I had joked with my girlfriends that they would be jealous of my "new, perky ones" and they had laughed that indeed they would. I was in the process of getting the desired and promised result. With the final surgery I would have upright and perfectly shaped "breasts." I would look like me in clothes, no bigger. Maybe better, we joked. Humour—it helps.

What most people cannot imagine is that when you have a bilateral mastectomy, all you are left with is the skin and two incisions that extend completely across the width of where the breasts were. There are, as we say in medicine, no normal anatomical landmarks. When you have a mastectomy, everything is gone, including nipple and areola. And indeed it is not a pretty sight. Although I had gotten used to the new me, it was clear that it was not normal.

I was thrilled to have almost all the reconstructive surgery behind me, with its pain and impairment. For the most part the temporary expanders were comfortable but I was constantly aware of them. The implants sit underneath the muscle on the chest wall. And being somewhat thin, with not a whole lot of body fat, I could actually feel the top edge of the implant on one side. I could see the pectoral muscles ripple after I exercised, which gave my chest an odd appearance. After all, there is no breast on top of the muscles, as normal people have.

Sleep now found me rolling onto my stomach, which I had not done for months. But the discomfort often woke me; I know now that it may never be entirely comfortable to lie that way.

There were days when the muscles felt stretched and sore. If I carried my computer and a carry-on bag, as I always do when I travel, I would have a day of severe chest-wall pain. The pectoral muscles, particularly on the right side where the cancer had been, remained extremely tight and sore. Dr. Lipa told me that likely I would always have an awareness of them being there. And while Stacy and I continue to work to stretch and release the muscles, I imagine it will never be as it was before. Then again, nothing will ever be as it was before.

While I was getting used to my physical appearance, every time I stepped out of the shower my image in the mirror would catch my eye and stop me, if only for a moment. How odd these smooth chest mounds, as the doctors called them, actually looked! The nasty red scars were fading. As a friend and colleague reminded me, the finished product was for a limited viewing audience. And that was entirely true. But when Jenna and I went to a spa together to use a gift certificate someone had sent, I received odd glances from other women in the communal change room. After all, I looked like Barbie! And Barbie, just like Ken, is not anatomically correct. Still, for all the oddness of how these new breasts looked, I began to understand how some women, sick of all the surgeries and interventions, would not go back for what I affectionately called the final artwork.

Joan still had the exchange surgery to do, and the artwork could not be done at the same time. She suggested that I allow six months after the next and final surgery for healing of all the incisions before going back to finish up. She stressed that she felt it was important to complete the cosmetic work. With Joan's opinion in mind, and my increasing awareness that I felt odd about my breasts, I met with her to discuss what my choices were.

The areolae seemed an easy decision, a no-brainer—of course I wanted them. Tattooing or stencilling an area is what is recommended. But when Joan asked me how large and what colour I wanted, I was stopped in my tracks by the burden of the decision. Another question was placement of the stencils. I looked at her and said, "I just want to look normal—not too dark, not too light; not too high, not too low." Like Goldilocks, I wanted "just right"—but what was just right?

Joan told me that the average size of an areola is 42 millimetres. This seemed to be more information than I'd ever needed or wanted to know. She suggested I go home and cut out a circle of that diameter and try it on for size and location. I flashed back to playing with cut-out dolls when I was a little girl, trying the different outfits on my cardboard dolls. Another suggestion was to look at paint chips or lipstick colours and find one I liked. I could just see myself at a cosmetic counter at Holt Renfrew: instead of trying out test colours on the back of my hand, I could whip out an implant.

Then we got to the discussion about the nipple itself. Truth was, I enjoyed the fact that I never needed to wear a bra—after all, these breasts were eternally perky and smooth. A nipple would be visible in a fitted shirt. Now I wasn't so sure I wanted them!

I asked women who had had nipple reconstruction to show me their results. As a physician, when I examine women with reconstruction I am paying close attention to possible recurrence of cancer along the scar line; I never really look at them from a cosmetic viewpoint. Now it was clear to me that the results would be subtle and I decided that I did in fact want to finish up. However, we ran into a technical stumbling block.

When skin is transplanted from one part of the body to another, the most common locations to choose from are the ear lobe or the labia. The skin from these areas is the least likely to flatten out or be rejected. But I have very small ear lobes (which I had not realized), and one had been made even smaller by an accident early on in my career. I was wearing earrings at the office one day when a small child got her finger caught in my earring loop as I examined her. The earring ripped through my lobe, and in having the lobe repaired part of it was lost. Who knew then I might one day need it! And so the ear lobe was not an option: too small, not enough skin.

The idea of using the labia, truth be known, just didn't sit right with me. Joan offered me a third site, which was the base of my fourth toe. But I recalled an earlier visit to Dr. McCready, who does a lot of foot surgery for melanoma, when he told me that skin on the foot often does not heal well. Now Joan confirmed that there might be an issue with healing. I thought about it for a while but did not feel it was worth the risk. I love to exercise, speed walk, run and snowshoe, ski. My feet were too important to my mental health and I was not ready to jeopardize them.

Joan suggested that we try avoiding a skin transplant alto- gether and simply tattoo the central area of the stencil a little darker, but in the end there seemed to be enough skin left at the end of the incisions; they might offer up just enough to get a cosmetic result. After the transplant was done, it would be important to avoid any shearing on the chest wall, and so I would have to allow time for healing, which meant no exer- cise. When the transplants had healed, I would have to come back yet again to tattoo them and make them blend in. She reminded me they would be pale, since they were coming from regular skin. This was a lot to think about!

My secretary and friend Barb, who had had the reconstruc- tion surgery two years prior, was ready to have her final sur- gery. We decided that when I was finally ready we would book together, back to back. The procedure is done under a local anesthetic rather than a general. We would make a party of it—go together for the procedure and then go for lunch!

And so, with the "final artwork" procedure planned, it seemed to me the signal that all this would eventually be over. But I knew it would never be truly over. There was no absolute reassurance for me. I was going to have to learn to live with uncertainty.

TWENTY-ONE

Run your own race

I often lecture about balance and wellbeing. As part of that speech I talk about accountability. So when it came time to think about doing a documentary about my experience with breast cancer, I realized that first and foremost it was myself I had to be accountable to.

I thought for a long time about why I wanted to do the documentary. Initially, after the press release was made and I was inundated with well-wishers, flowers and phone calls, I just wanted to be left alone. To smoulder and be angry and cope as best I could—alone, not under the glare of the public spotlight. The reality was that the physical effects of cancer treatment—the various side effects, the feeling of my body becoming a toxic waste dump—are only part of why this disease is so difficult. The emotional impact—learning who I was stripped of my career, watching my family cope as best they could, living in fear for my life—was harrowing and often devastating. This disease was changing me. Yet in all my years of caring for patients, the emphasis had always been on the medical side of things. Few people in the medical community speak publicly about the emotional impact, the sense of fear, aloneness and anger, the jumble of emotions endured by almost anyone facing a life-threatening illness.

I felt that I had a story to tell. It was clear that I did not have all the "right" answers—having cancer was no easier for me, a doctor, than for anyone else, although to many it appeared that it was. After all, there I was, week after week, on air, making it look easy. As I often joked, I gave cancer a bad name. I did my best to challenge the common assumption that cancer is an inevitable death sentence. As my friend Rob Buckman would point out, cancer is a word and not a sentence. I did cancer right, whatever that might mean. I did my best to carry on a normal life, continuing to work on air and finding a new career as a medical columnist for the *Globe and Mail*. But when it came to the treatment itself and the challenges of learning to live with breast cancer, I was very clear that I didn't want people to think I had the inside track. As knowledgeable as I may be, I am not an oncologist. The decisions I made were personal and unique to my case. What I wanted to talk about was not so much the science or the medical advances, but my personal story. Our story. What had struck me when I left the set of Vicki Gabereau's show was that so many people who waited to talk to me said I was the first to validate their fears, to say out loud that it was okay to be angry, it was okay to be bald. I did not (and do not) believe my family's story is all that different from many other stories out there. But if it would be helpful to other women and their families, as I believed it might be, then it was worth going on air nationally and speaking candidly. It was not and is not that I am any different from anyone else. What was different was that I had a platform.

Bobby and I sat down to talk about it. I wasn't sure I actually wanted to do this, and he wasn't sure we should either. But it was clear that *we* were making this decision: I could not tell the story without my family agreeing to do this, without my friends agreeing. It was also clear that I could not censor anyone. My children, my family, all had to be free to speak their truth.

Bobby initially pointed out that I would be talking about the mastectomy and reconstruction, deeply personal decisions that we had struggled to make. I was worried about the exposure for my children and how much this might invade their privacy. We debated these concerns for a while, but ultimately it was Bobby who asked the questions that made us both shift our thinking: Why, he asked, if one in nine women has breast cancer, are there so few bald women walking around? Why was I one of the first he had seen? Wearing a wig, trying to fit into what our society sees as normal, yet being isolated by cancer— this seemed to be the norm. So often he had felt isolated during this ordeal, the girls felt isolated, and clearly I felt that way much of the time. Sharing our story might indeed be helpful.

The filming began to gather what was happening. Although we had filmed some of what we had been through, and there was lots of footage of me at work and on *Vicki,* here was a production crew dedicated to more or less living with all of us and telling our story. We accumulated hours and hours of footage.

When CTV agreed to give me free rein, for which I will always be grateful, they introduced me to Gordon Henderson of 90th Parallel, an independent production company. Although Gordon and I had not worked together on the *Balance* set for my daytime show, he had done the nighttime *Balance* specials hosted by Valerie Pringle. A kind and thoughtful man, he had won many Geminis and understood a side of the business that

I did not. As executive producer, he would oversee that business side. He met with me to talk about the making of the documentary. He listened carefully to me and understood quickly that I didn't want a documentary about the science and medicine behind breast cancer, that this was to be a personal story. In turn, Gordon introduced me to Mary Anne Alton, who would be my co-producer. Mary Anne just got me and got what I wanted to do, or at least what I thought I wanted to do. In retrospect, I see that I had no clue how difficult it would be.

Mary Anne—along with Robert Holmes, the director of photography, and Brent Haliskie, my sound man—became part of my life, our life. One day I sat down with them and spent four hours narrating the events as they had happened. That footage would ultimately form the backbone of the documentary.

To bring viewers right into the experience, we began filming events in real time, taking the cameras into appointments and the surgeries that followed. But it was clear that we also had to recreate the very beginning. Mary Anne and I talked a lot about that, and because we believed that many women did not really understand what a mammogram was about, we saw this as an opportunity to show and explain the technical end of it. My doctors agreed to let the cameras in as we recreated those first medical appointments, and they also agreed to be interviewed for the documentary.

I could not imagine how emotionally difficult it would be to revisit many of the issues and to look at them once they were on film. There were times when Mary Anne, Robert, Brent and I all wanted to cry, times when it was just too painful. After a while I didn't notice the camera or any of the crew. They became part of the background noise as I tried to get through to the other side.

After the hysterectomy, but before the final reconstructive surgery, we agreed that we would go to California to see Dr. Susan Love. Susan and I had been in contact with each other from the very beginning. Her advice had been conservative; she had not been in favour of chemotherapy, and was certainly not in favour of the bilateral mastectomy. I had chosen to be quite aggressive, and with the chemo and surgeries now behind me, I was well enough to go visit her. Dr. Love agreed that we could come with a crew.

I was an emotional wreck going to see her. A world expert had given me the benefit of her thoughts and time, and I had not followed her course of advice. I was anxious—not anxious that she would disapprove, but anxious that I had made the wrong choices. Although I had promised myself not to look back, that was exactly what I was doing. Second-guessing.

As I walked up to see her, the camera crew recording it all, I was focused only on her, our unfolding conversation and the incredible anxiety and second thoughts I was having. We reviewed what had happened and all the choices I had made. She was calm and reassuring, reinforcing her position once again that there was no single right answer. *The* answer did not exist; there were only choices between courses of action that are thought to be equivalent in terms of long-term outcome. I told her that I was worried I had been too aggressive, perhaps done too much. My decisions, carefully thought out and informed by consultations with experts, had perhaps been emotional. I did not believe they had been knee-jerk decisions, or irrational, but perhaps emotional.

She looked at me and asked, "In the absence of a clear answer, what else is there but emotion?" Emotion was fine, she said, understandable and perhaps the only way to make decisions when we're presented with uncertain choices and no clear answers. With time I would stop being anxious, she reminded me; days and then years would go by and I would realize that I was no longer thinking about cancer every waking moment, and then I would not think about it at all. It was a process, a process I could not rush.

I knew she was right. From coping with Jason's death, I had learned that second-guessing and self-doubt are a form of grief and mourning. And like the journey of coping with his death, this too would take its own course. I knew there would be a time when the anxiety would not walk in front of me, but beside me, and eventually behind me. Only time would let me heal from the physical and emotional scars.

With our conversation finished, I walked for hours trying to digest it all. I tried to tell myself, once and for all, that I had done what I believed was best for me at the time and that there was no turning back. I had to let it go. I had no choice but to let it go. With that knowledge in hand, I flew home, ready to face the last of the major surgeries.

The final surgery was the removal of the expanders and the placement of the implants. After this, only the cosmetic work would remain, to be done six months later. The camera crew was with me every step of the way. I really was not nervous. It was the last stop on a very long journey. But Susan and Renee were with me, as they had been for every surgery, and my now extended family of Mary Anne, Robert and Brent were with me. Bobby and I arrived yet again at Toronto General Hospital at 6 a.m. for what seemed like a familiar routine. I needed this one last surgery to be over. I needed this behind me. I could almost imagine a life not dictated by surgeries and chemotherapy, endless doctors' appointments, nausea and side effects from medications. As I was being put to sleep, Joan said to me, "Think a happy thought." I remember thinking that I simply wanted this to be over, but as I drifted off I saw myself walking down the aisle at Matthew's wedding. I was serene and calm and I realized my happy thought was one of life, being alive with Matt on such a special day in his future. He was, at that time, only 10 years old, but I knew what my psyche was saying to me.

The surgery itself was successful and initially seemed to have been uneventful. As before, I had practised my sit-ups, ready to make sure that no one touched me when the elephants had once again taken a seat on my chest. The next day, when my family doctor and close friend Vivien came to see me, she immediately noticed that the anesthetist had knocked off the top of my bottom tooth. I just did not seem to get along well with anesthesia. I went home the next day, my sister Zozzie and brother-in-law David there to care for me, and my wonderful support group of friends at hand.

Within 24 hours, though, I was dehydrated and had spiked a fever. Bobby and David rushed me back to the hospital. Confused and delirious, I awoke in the same room that I had been discharged from, without much memory of what had happened. I remember waking and feeling hot and sick, furious and confused, all at the same time. Could this not just be over? Could we not put this all behind us?

With an antibiotic drip and fluid rehydrating me, I picked up fairly quickly and once again was able to go home. But, ever mindful of the pectoral muscles that once again had been lifted from my chest to allow removal of the expanders and exchange of the implants, I promised to be a good patient to allow full recovery. The elephants were indeed back sitting on my chest, the pain all too familiar.

With that final discharge, the worst of my surgeries were now behind me and I could actually think about a return-to-work date. It seemed impossible that I could actually allow myself to think about returning to work, returning to my career. As I said in the documentary, I looked forward to getting up and complaining about going to work rather than getting up and complaining about being sick.

The documentary was almost ready to be cut. But it was time for my friends and family to speak for the cameras. Mary Anne interviewed Bobby and the girls. I was not present for those interviews. I did not want them censored in any way, and told them to speak freely and candidly.

My girlfriends talked about how I had shut them out and only with their persistence had I learned to let them in. Learned to accept their kindness and learned to stop always needing to be in control. They talked about distracting me through the surgeries, trying to make me laugh and to take us all away emotionally to another place.

Gwen, my first mentor, came to be filmed. She talked about how this would change me forever, in some ways for the better. She talked about seeing the future and how this would change my relationships with my patients and change me as a doctor, a person, a wife, a friend and a mother.

Bobby spoke of the public perception of me sailing through all this, how this perception was not the reality. His perception was of a woman who woke at night fearful, wondering if she would be there to see her children get married, wondering if she would be there to see the birth of her grandchildren. He was the only one who talked about me dying. The only one to say it out loud. He talked about how difficult I could be, how sick I had been, how horrible this had been for all of them.

And he laughed about my recovery, about my hair beginning to come back in and how he could no longer see the glow of the fluorescent clock off my shiny bald head.

And my daughters. My daughters talked about how in some ways my breast cancer was the best thing that had ever happened to our relationship. I knew what Jenna was talking about when she said this but it was very hard to hear. I cried when I saw that on air. I knew that she was saying that while I had always been emotionally available to her I had not always been physically there. That many of my career decisions had been selfish and had affected them.

Amanda spoke of what it felt like the day she was invested as a prefect. What it felt like to know that I could be there if I tried, no matter how sick I was. It had given us both hope that I could make this go away with medication and surgery, and be there for all her important life events. She talked about how my values of work and family and self—the balance of my values—had changed. She meant that I had learned a painful lesson about investing the time and the emotions synchronously in my family values. I applauded my daughters' bravery and honesty, as painful as their words were for me. They were speaking of true, difficult life lessons. I had learned the lesson that I am here now, and now is what counts. This is my time, their time, our time, and it is not to be wasted or treated lightly. I was grateful to the part of having this disease that had made it possible for me to learn these lessons now, before it was too late.

With the release of the documentary pending, I wrote a first-person piece for the *Globe and Mail* to coincide with the release; it summarized much of what I felt during the treatment. I spoke candidly about the changes that had happened to me and to my family and what a journey this had been. The piece went to press that Saturday with pictures of me and the kids. There was no turning back now.

CTV released a press notice about the documentary. It read as follows:

For Immediate Release (Oct. 5, 2005)

—Doctor Becomes Patient in Emotional CTV Special—
Run Your Own Race: Dr. Marla's Journey With Breast Cancer, Oct. 15—Dr. Shapiro's own emotional journey timed with National Breast Cancer Awareness Month—

Toronto, ON (October 5, 2005)—She's on TV every day discussing healthy living and lifestyle but without warning last summer, CTV's Dr. Marla Shapiro went from doctor to patient after being diagnosed with breast cancer. Since then, she's been running the race of her life, enduring a rollercoaster wave of emotion along the way. Now Dr. Marla is telling her private story, from diagnosis to recovery, in Run Your Own Race: Dr. Marla's Journey With Breast Cancer. The one-hour special, timed to coincide with the midpoint of National Breast Cancer Awareness Month, airs Saturday, Oct. 15 at 7 p.m. ET (check local listings) on CTV.

To viewers, Dr. Marla is best known as both host of CTV's daytime series *Balance: Television for Living Well* and as medical consultant for CTV News. In the special, Shapiro herself takes viewers on a yearlong journey, from the mammogram that changed her life forever to the recovery that lies ahead. Coming face-to-face with fear, anxiety and uncertainty, Dr. Shapiro honestly and openly describes how cancer affected not just herself, but her friends, family and the general public.

"As CTV's medical consultant it has been a privilege to be invited into the homes of Canadian viewers to interpret the medical news of the day," said Dr. Shapiro. "It's now an honour to invite you into my home to take this journey with me as I run my own race."

"This experience gave me the opportunity to share what I learned," adds Dr. Shapiro. "It is a natural extension of my role as a family physician and educator."

"Dr. Marla Shapiro has turned the tables around so that we the viewers can see her as a patient trying to get the answers, rather than a doctor who has all the answers," said Susanne Boyce, President of Programming and Chair of the CTV Media Group. "We admire her for her courage in sharing this experience with us as she deals with such a personal battle."

Combining clips of Dr. Shapiro's medical team with those of her husband, children, friends and television peers, the special focuses as much on her emotional conflict as it does on her clinical diagnosis and treatment. From her original mammogram to numerous consultations with physicians, Dr. Shapiro's journey depicts the life-altering decisions made about treatments for which there are no clear answers. After multiple surgical interventions and an arduous run of chemotherapy, Dr. Shapiro makes the difficult decision to have a bilateral mastectomy and reconstructive surgery.

Throughout her battle, Dr. Shapiro is in continual contact with world-renowned breast cancer specialist and friend Dr. Susan Love. After her chemotherapy, viewers travel with Dr. Shapiro to California as she meets with Dr. Love to discuss what she's been through and how to navigate her future decisions.

"I am so grateful to Marla Shapiro for going beyond the usual feel good breast cancer special to show women that often what we don't know is greater than what we do know," says Dr. Susan Love, MD MBA, a world-renowned author and one of the founding mothers of the breast cancer advocacy movement. "And finding the right answer is difficult."

After her visit to California, Dr. Shapiro proceeds with reconstructive surgery. Cameras follow her into the hospital room as she prepares for yet another surgery. With warm wishes from her friends, Dr. Shapiro says "ciao" as she is taken into the operating room for the last time.

The documentary is also very fitting for Canadian viewers as October is National Breast Cancer Awareness Month (NBCAM). 2005 marks more than 20 years that NBCAM has educated women about early breast cancer detection, diagnosis and treatment.

Originally from Montreal, Dr. Shapiro completed medical school at McGill University. She is a Certificant of the College of Family Physicians of Canada and a Specialist in Community Medicine as recognized by her Fellowship from the Royal College of Physicians and Surgeons of Canada.

She is an Associate Professor in the Department of Family and Community Medicine at the University of Toronto and is in full time private practice. Dr. Shapiro has been published and lectures frequently. Dr. Shapiro is a spokesperson for the Princess Margaret Hospital Breast Cancer Survivorship Program. Dr. Shapiro is the recipient of the 2005 NAMS (North American Menopause Society) Media Award for her work in expanding the knowledge and understanding of menopause. Dr. Shapiro is also a weekly contributor on *Canada AM* and the medical consultant for CTV *Newsnet*. Dr. Shapiro is also the host of *Balance: Television for Living Well,* the daily half-hour show that gives viewers health and lifestyle information.

The Friday before the *Globe* article ran and the show aired, through the magic of satellite I was interviewed in every market and every province across our country. There appeared to be a lot of interest in our story. We went to air with hundreds of thousands watching and received many, many e-mails from viewers. As with my appearance on *The Vicki Gabereau Show,* the response was startling and reassuring—there had been good reason to tell this story. I was grateful that it seemed helpful to many. I was grateful to my family, my children and friends for bearing with me and for allowing the story to be told. In 2006, the documentary would receive accolades from another source when it won the gold REMI at the Houston International Film Festival.

Weeks after the documentary first aired, I flew to New York to interview Melissa Etheridge about the launch of her new CD. Jordan Schwartz, my executive producer for *Balance,* and the former executive producer of *Canada AM* who had brought me to CTV, was now the force behind *eTalk Daily.* Although I was not an entertainment reporter, he felt I was the right person to do this interview. And though I was there to talk about her music, it was clear that I was the interviewer because we had shared parallel experiences. We talked about her becoming an accidental and reluctant activist. I related on a personal level as she described feelings that echoed so many of my own. Neither one of us would have chosen the path but we both felt committed to taking our experiences forward. We talked about the name of her CD, *The Road Less Traveled*. I knew exactly what that road meant to me and how it was not so different from my documentary, *Run Your Own Race*. The interview ended with her saying, "I could talk to you for hours." I felt exactly the same way. Celebrity, entertainer, singer or doctor, we are both women. In the end, we have endured similar experiences, with similar emotions, but our paths are still unique to us.

As much as I did not want breast cancer to define me, it has indeed refined me. I think that my experience, like every other cancer patient's, has changed me in ways both perceptible and imperceptible. It is clear that I am not the same woman who walked into mammography the morning of Friday, August 13, 2004. It is clear that because of who I am and what I do, I can never be fully reassured that the cancer is gone forever. And while I cannot rush time forward and walk down the aisle with any of my children, what I can do is live each and every day mindfully.

So how have I changed? In many ways I am the same, juggling a zillion work balls and loving the return to my busy schedule. But in so many other ways I am different. The only word I can think of is *mindful*. I am so much more conscious of the decisions I make, of my family, my children and how I choose to live my life. My children would tell you my values have changed—perhaps they were already far wiser than their mother, who had to learn how to match her emotional commitments with her time commitments.

I am no different than any other man or woman or family struggling to cope with a chronic illness. I have done it a bit more publicly. To those of you who say I have inspired you with my so-called courage, I would tell you it is the opposite: you have inspired me with your stories and your own fights. It doesn't take courage to fight when there is no other option. But it has taken courage to look at me, at who I was, who I am and the choices I have made.

People ask me all the time how I live with the uncertainty. I often smile at the question because it suggests that the person asking doesn't also live with uncertainty. The fact is that we all do, each and every one of us. The difference is that my uncertainty has a name. It is called breast cancer. But having a name does not lend any certainty to its outcome. Breast cancer, like any chronic illness, can begin to assume an identity and then, if you let it, a life of its own. Unchallenged, unhealthy beliefs become your reality if you let them. That inevitably leads to fear and anxiety, and just being, well, off balance. Yet with time, as Susan Love pointed out to me, an obsessive fear about uncertainty, about "what if," will usually disappear and become less of a focus.

While it is tempting to succumb to the angst of what if, it is far better to deal with what is. And the what is, for me, is that I am here. Now. I am here. I hope to be a woman who dies with breast cancer, not because of breast cancer.

I have been told that cancer is like a gift wrapped in barbed wire. For me, that has been the case. After the pain of the treatment, the fear and irrational moments, I have had a chance to meet with me and learn a little more about me. And in knowing who I am, I can only be a better mother, friend, wife, doctor—a better person. I am grateful for that knowledge and that clarity.

And so it has gone, this year in my life, this year that has helped to shape who I am today and who I am yet to become. Some say this is a journey, a journey with, through and ultimately beyond. I thank you for letting me share the journey with you.

PART FOUR

THE JURY SPEAKS

TWENTY-TWO

Jenna's story

I have always been a firm believer that everything happens for a reason. There is never a good reason for anyone to have to fight cancer, but in our family we deal with unfortunate circumstances with a positive attitude. Losing my brother Jason to sudden infant death syndrome was the hardest thing we ever had to go through as a family. Although it was hard to stay positive, we did, and a year later we got the biggest gift from God, my brother Matthew. Matthew made us realize that everything happens for a reason and he makes me remember every day how lucky we are even though we have had to deal with extremely hard times. When my mom was diagnosed with breast cancer I knew that we would get through this, just as we have gotten through everything else.

My mom isn't the average mom. My mom is "Dr. Marla." Over the past 13 years she has become a woman not only whom I admire, but whom the rest of the world aspires to be like. While I was growing up, and to this day, people would stop us on the street and ask if we are sisters; now people stop her everywhere to tell her how amazing she is. It is a wonder that it hasn't gone to her head. Some people may not believe that and say that it is not possible to remain in reality when you live a life like my mother's, but being her daughter, the daughter who looks just like her, I can say that this is true. Maybe it is her twelve hundred jobs that keep her down-to-earth, maybe it is us, her family, or maybe it is my indescribably loud voice that doesn't let her escape reality for a minute. It has always amazed me how even in the toughest situations she is concerned about everyone else before herself. This battle has been no different.

It was the end of the summer in 2004, when I was looking through a clutter of papers in the kitchen, that I found some information on a core biopsy. Although I haven't always been the "brains" in the family, I knew something was going on. A few days later, my mom met Amanda and me at the hairdresser's with an ice pack on her chest and a look of uneasiness in her eyes. Amanda was in the chair getting her hair cut and my mom was sitting in the next room. I immediately went over to her and asked what was going on. She told me that we would have to sit down as a family and talk. Right then I knew I would hear that my mother was fighting cancer. As I tried to hold in my fear that these words would later be spoken to me, I went on with my day, acting as if nothing was wrong in order not to upset my sister. I kept seven o'clock open that night, knowing that if I didn't the conversation would be put off and I would be in the dark a little bit longer. As I anxiously awaited my dad's return from work, I dreaded the conversation that was about to take place, and hoped that my assumptions were wrong. When I heard my dad open the garage, I took my brother upstairs to play Gamecube, which I knew would entertain him for a while. My mom, dad, sister and I sat down together downstairs and I heard the words that I had known were coming all day. Mom told us that she had breast cancer but that it was nothing to worry about because they had caught it early and things were going to be okay. As my sister sat on the opposite side of the room with my dad, she looked at me in confusion, as if wondering why I did not seem surprised. I looked at my mom and said, "I knew it," and told her how I had put the pieces together. I did not want to be kept in the dark for a second longer, I said; I wanted her to let me know everything as soon as she herself knew.

That week my dad was leaving for China for two weeks and the rest of us were going to Chicago for a few days to spend some time together. My mom received a phone call towards the end of the trip and, although she didn't tell me about it right away, I could tell she had received news that she didn't want to hear. A little while later she let me know that she would be having an operation to remove the cancerous area. A week after our return from Chicago I was leaving to start my second year at the University of Western Ontario in London. The surgery was scheduled for a Friday, so I told my mom that I would be home that evening to spend the weekend with her. I was scared. This was no longer a little issue that they had "caught early." This was something that I knew would affect our lives. My dad called from China every day and I missed him more than ever. I could hear the fright in his voice, although he kept telling me that he was fine. All I wanted was for us all to be together and confide in one another, but that was not going to happen right away—my dad would not return from China until after I had left for school.

All my mother's friends were more than willing to take her to appointments and sit with her through them at the hospital but I decided that I would be that friend to her for as long as

I could. At the end of August, Amanda and I took her to an appointment with her surgeon. I remember sitting in the cancer ward waiting room. There were so many women. Some had hair and some didn't; some looked very ill and some didn't. I couldn't help but wonder how my mom's body would react to the cancer. Would she have to go through radiation or chemotherapy? Would she lose her hair? Would her breasts have to be removed? And, worst of all, would the cancer spread? I had so many questions and there were so few answers. While we were sitting in the waiting room a woman across from us looked at my mom and asked her if she was Dr. Marla. It was a tough position. We were not interested in the world finding out about this, gossiping about it, but it was inevitable that someone would recognize my mother. I found it hard to believe that someone would have the nerve to ask such a question in that setting. People were curious about what was happening with the famous Dr. Marla and I was wondering what was happening to my mom. When she went into the examining room, my sister and I stayed in the waiting room. I kept asking myself, *Haven't we been through enough—and what have we done to deserve this?* Deep down I knew they were unanswerable questions.

A few days later, I drove my mom to the hospital for an MRI. On the way, she began to cry. It was the first time that I saw her true emotions about everything that was going on. It was the first time that I heard her utter the words "I'm scared." She began to let all of her fears about her disease come out into the real world, out to me, her eldest daughter. Fears about not being around for my wedding, or around to be a grandmother. Her fears of not being able to see my sister become the amazing woman that she is destined to be and fears of not seeing her little boy grow to be a man. It was the first time that I felt it was normal to have the feelings I was having. It gave me a sense of relief to know that she could confide in me and that she wasn't afraid to tell me the truth. I held in my tears to be strong for her.

At this point, my mom and dad had decided that we would keep quiet about my mother's diagnosis. But my mom respected the fact that I would need to talk to someone, and encouraged me to tell my lifelong best friend, Cheri Glina. The only problem was that Cheri had moved to Israel for the year. The person who knew my family better than anyone else, the person I felt most comfortable talking to, the person who could always make me feel better was now so far away. I called her and confided in her and she talked me through it—as she always had. She confirmed everything that I already knew. She told me that my mom is the strongest person she knows and that there was no doubt in her mind that she would get through this. I realized that my main concern was that I would be at school while all this was happening.

Shortly after that conversation, an event happened that confirmed my fears. Early in the week of my mom's scheduled surgery, I was planning what time to leave London on the Friday. Then I got a call from my mother. From the sound of her voice I knew that I had been kept in the dark. This was not the voice of my happy mom. This was the voice of my mom calling to tell me that she had just gotten out of surgery. I didn't know what to feel: relieved that the surgery was over or angry that she hadn't told me about the changed date. I had taken the call while in a room with two friends who had no idea about my mom's cancer, so I walked out into the hall, finished the conversation with her and then broke down. I didn't want her to hear me cry. Although her reasons for not telling me were in my best interests, I was still so upset. I wondered if there were other things I wasn't being told. My sister called later that afternoon to see how I was doing because my mom had told her I was very upset with her. I immediately called my mom at the hospital to apologize and to assure her that I wasn't upset with her, I was just confused and scared. She understood, as I knew she would. My Aunt Wendy was in the hospital with her when I called. Wendy and I have a very close relationship, so she came on the phone and reassured me that everything was fine and that my mom was doing great. It was hard for me because I was hours away and all I had was the sound of my mom's voice, which was tired and quiet. Not being able to see her made everything so much worse. We spoke numerous times that night and I told her that I would be home that Friday afternoon.

When I got home a few days later my mom was the first person I saw. All I wanted to do was give her a hug but I was afraid that I would hurt her. She unbuttoned her shirt and showed me the swelling and the bruising. Her entire chest was completely black and blue and around her armpits was severely swollen. It looked so painful and uncomfortable that it was hard for me to look at, and harder still to know what to say. With her shirt closed again, she looked like the same amazing person I had always known. She walked into the kitchen and went on with her day, just like her old self.

When I came home over the next couple of weekends, it seemed there was always more bad news. My mom would talk about it freely with me but she had to speak quietly because Matthew was still unaware of what was going on. One night, after my mom had received some upsetting news, I was standing with her in the kitchen as she was teaching me to make one of her salad dressings when my dad walked in. He saw the strained look on her face and asked what was wrong. The only thing she found that she could respond with was, "I have cancer. That's what's wrong." Later that night I was checking my e-mail while Matt was playing Nintendo. There was a message from my mom, an encouraging message that reminded me she was the same person I had always known and that she would beat this with a positive attitude. As I was responding to the e-mail Matt came up to the computer and I told him to go back and sit on the couch. He looked at me and asked, "Why? Because Mom has cancer?" I was shocked. Right away I asked him what he had just said and where he had heard that, but he just responded with a shrug and an "I dunno" and went back to playing his game. I knew it was time my parents told him something. This very smart nine-year-old knew exactly what was going on and he was scared.

I went back to school after that weekend, and early the next week got a call from my mom. She had just come from the doctor's office and wanted me to know that the doctor had recommended chemotherapy. In most cases, this would have been unappealing news, but I knew from the sound of her voice that it was exactly the opposite. She sounded at peace with it. From the information she had given me about how they had reached the decision, it came to me that this was the "best" bad news we had heard since day one. I was a little scared, but I knew that she would get through it and I would be right by her side as her friend, her confidante and, of course, her daughter.

Matthew was told soon enough. Mom would have to stop working, which meant that she would be home almost all the time. This was going to be the biggest change of all for the rest of the family. My mom not working is an anomaly—she was never the mom who was home at lunchtime. That was never a problem for any of us; it was just the way life was. When I was younger I was so excited on those rare days when I would see her car in the driveway at the end of a school day. Now Matthew was going see her car in the driveway at the end of every school day. Would this be a good thing or a bad thing? Could she be a stay-at-home mom for a while, looking at it as a chance to relax and watch her son grow up for a few months, or would she go nuts from staying at home all the time? All these questions ran through my head, but I knew that my Dr. Marla would find her balance at home.

I came home again after I knew about the decision to start chemotherapy. At this point she had already cut down on work time and was home to spend some time with me. There were numerous times during that weekend when my mom and I would go into the big closet in her room, close the door and talk about life. We talked about everything that was going on in my life and my concerns, and about everything that was on her mind and her concerns. It was really nice to know that we could sit down and have a conversation about important things or nothing at all and that she had nowhere to run to. I didn't have to schedule a time to talk with her; she had all the time in the world to talk to me. In my heart, I felt that the cancer diagnosis might have been the end of something bad and the beginning of something good. I felt that the battle would be hard, but at the same time it would somehow bring my mom and me closer together.

A few weeks later, during one of our phone calls, she told me that she would be starting chemotherapy on that Tuesday, the Tuesday before the Thanksgiving weekend. She told me that she had lots of people who had offered to go with her and that it would be fine. She said that she would call me after and let me know how it went. At the end of that first day she called me but she didn't really want to talk about it. She had also told me earlier that week that she was going to go public so that people would know what was going on rather than having them talk about what they thought was going on. The Tuesday that she started chemo was the day that the news of her cancer would come out to the rest of the world. She told me to watch the 11 o'clock news and she sent me the articles that were in the newspapers. As I read one article I was appalled that it made mention of my brother Jason's death. My mom was on the phone with me while I read the article because she knew that when I read it I was going to be very upset. As always, she was right. It didn't make much sense to me. Was it not enough that my mom had cancer and now everyone knew? Why did everyone have to know about Jason as well? I was extremely annoyed.

For the rest of the week the phone was ringing off the hook. People had heard on the radio, from the paper and through word of mouth. It was hard having everyone calling but nice to know that people cared. My mom and I spoke numerous times in the days after that first chemo treatment. One of the things we spoke about was my having some friends from Montreal come to visit me that weekend. I didn't realize that she would be feeling ill that weekend. Once she told me, I immediately revoked the question and sent her an e-mail to apologize for having asked at all. The next thing I knew the phone was ringing: it was my mom, wanting me to know that she hated saying no to me because she didn't want her cancer to affect my life. She didn't want me to have to change my plans because she was going to be sick that weekend. I knew right then that she would deal with this whole battle as her doctor-self who always handles everything: she was more interested in taking care of her family (the "patients") than herself. That is what doctors do—or at least what this doctor does. She did not see herself as a patient.

I called my friends and told them that it just wasn't a good time and maybe we could see each other another time. I didn't mention the cancer at all. But the day before I was going home I got a call from my friends in Montreal; they said they were coming to see me after all and would be staying at a hotel. I was so excited—it was exactly what I needed. I went home to see my mom and I told her what their plan was. She told me that they should stay at our house because she was feeling fine and my friends should not stay in a hotel no matter what. But by Friday night she wasn't feeling well and she stayed home while the rest of our family went to my Aunty Wendy's for dinner. She still managed to make sure that by the time we left for dinner she had a chocolate cake ready for my cousin Jesse; it had been his birthday earlier that week and chocolate cake was his favourite.

The next morning I woke up and went to see my mom. She was in bed. She couldn't move and could hardly speak. She tried telling me how she felt. She said it was so hard to believe that she felt this way because the day before she had felt only nauseated and tired. I let her rest and went to get into bed with my sister. She was sleeping, but I really didn't want to be alone. We talked about what was going on and I asked if my mom had been like this before. She said that she hadn't. I went downstairs to talk to my dad. I told him how hard it was to see her like that. The house was very quiet and different. My dad made breakfast for my sister and me, and then my mom came downstairs. She lay down on the couch and watched some TV. I made her a cup of tea and remained quiet; she eventually fell asleep.

My friends called to tell me they were nearing the house, and though I was so excited to see them when they arrived, I took them quietly to my room and spent the afternoon talking and catching up. My mom didn't wake up until late in the afternoon. Of course my friends wanted to meet the famous Dr. Marla, so we went downstairs to see her. She pulled herself up to sitting, using the arm of the couch. She welcomed them to our home and seemingly without a second's thought invited them to stay with us for the weekend. We were all sitting in the den talking. I was sitting with my mom, holding her hand, and my friends were sitting on the opposite couch. I had feared that my mom would say something about the cancer, because she was very open about it. I was not worried because it made me uncomfortable (in fact, I liked that she spoke about it), but I was worried because I had not spoken to my friends about it yet and I didn't want them to feel uncomfortable. I should have known not to worry—my mom did bring it up but she also spoke of it in a way that made no one feel uncomfortable. She talked about the benefits of cancer in terms of shopping! She told them that now she could buy things she would have never bought and she could tell herself it was okay because she had cancer. She was very funny and happy as always. The next thing I knew she was asking everyone what they wanted for dinner. We ordered sushi and pizza and had a huge dinner with my two friends from Montreal, two of my sister's friends, my parents and my brother, and we laughed the entire time. It felt so good to have dinner together and to see my mom smiling and laughing.

My friends spent the night and the next morning my mom appeared to be feeling much better. I told her that I was going to take my friends to my favourite breakfast place and she looked at me as if I were crazy. She told me to go wake up the girls and bring them down for breakfast because she had gone shopping for a big breakfast—bagels and cream cheese and tuna and every type of cheese you could imagine. She had baked cakes and cookies and it was a fantastic breakfast. I wasn't sure if she was really feeling better or just doing her best to make me feel better. While she sat with us, she really couldn't eat, and when she tried to do some work, she would find she couldn't sit for long and would end up back on the couch. Still, from the looks of things, she was getting used to being at home. She was cooking and baking and experimenting with foods, getting used to a slower-placed life. At the end of the weekend I went back to school. Once I got there, my anxiety hit me full force. It was so much easier to be home and see her, even if she was sick, than to be away.

Back at school I was talking to a friend of mine about my relationship with my mom. It was strange for me to hear someone say how nice it was that my mom and I were so close. The previous year, the majority of our conversations had been over e-mail and we spoke about once a week, if that. We were still very close, but not nearly as close as we had become. My friend expressed the opinion that the relationship between children and their parents becomes stronger with age. That was when I realized that it also becomes closer because of cancer. When I told my mom about this conversation, she seemed insulted. To me, this was not something to be upset about but rather something to feel great about. The way I saw it, if my mom had to have cancer, then we might as well grow stronger from it.

We had many conversations in the next few weeks and she told me that she would be losing her hair. One day she told me that she had cut it all off because it was hard to watch it fall out. Later that week, my mom sent a package to me through a friend who had been in Toronto. She said it was very important. I went to pick it up and found that it contained a box of chocolates and an envelope. Written on the envelope were the words "I love you—Part of the original me. Mama." Right then I knew what was inside, and my eyes began to fill up with tears. Just as I expected, there was a piece of her hair, tied with a pink ribbon. Once I saw the hair I could no longer control the tears. Also written on the envelope, in a circle with a star next to it, was "Get a flu shot!" The doctor in her wasn't going to disappear simply because she was a patient now. I called her while I cried—she told me not to be such a wimp! I passed the phone to my roommate, who told my mom how much she looked up to her. Being the woman that my mom is, she made sure not to make my roommate feel uncomfortable and responded by saying, "Why? Because I'm taller than you?" A typical answer from an atypical woman.

The most tragic and memorable part of this experience was a phone call that I received the day my mom lost her hair. She came home to an empty house: I was in London, my sister was at school, my dad was at work and my brother was at an after-school program. Losing her hair was harder than she'd anticipated. It wasn't so much the idea that she was going to be bald, because, as we all know, she was able to embrace that, but it was the fact that for the first time she would look sick, she would no longer be able to ignore how her life was changing. In order to adjust to the hair-loss process, she had cut it all off in stages. But that day it was completely gone. She sat in her study in tears and, instead of pretending that she was able to deal with it all, she called me. Matt would be home within a matter of minutes and she was scared to see how he would react. Even she was frightened by the look, so it was reasonable to expect a less-than-perfect reaction from him. As she let her tears out, Matt walked in from school around dinner time while I was on the phone. He said, "Mom, you're scaring me. Put on a hat." She was alone and had to deal with a frightened child when she was frightened herself. She put Matt on the phone as she tried to calm down, but when I heard his voice my tears were unstoppable. The best I could do was to tell him that Mommy needed lots of hugs and lots of love. When he asked why I was crying, I said that I missed them. This was when the whole London–Toronto bit took its toll.

Believe it or not, the first time I saw my mom without hair was on *The Vicki Gabereau Show*. It was bizarre and amazing all at the same time. I was so proud that I had a mother who didn't feel the need to hide the "stigma" of cancer when the reality is that so many women go through this and no one would know. After seeing the show I went home for the weekend with my boyfriend at the time. I was okay with the fact that my mom was bald, but as she mentioned numerous times, she was very concerned about making my boyfriend feel uncomfortable. Would he prefer that she wear her wig? she wondered. But why would she wear a wig at home when she hadn't worn one on national TV? I found that no one close to us had a problem with the fact that my mom preferred not to wear a wig; the wigs made her head sweat and itch. When my mom told me that some people (who didn't really know her) felt otherwise, I was disgusted. How could people judge her if they had never been through something like this? When I was home, I was glad to see that my mom was able to embrace the fact that she was bald, rather than dwell on it. She had the cutest beanie hats that she would wear around the house. We all agreed that her fuzzy orange fitted cap made her look like Dopey of the seven dwarfs!

The middle of my mom's chemotherapy brought us to November, and to my 20th birthday. I wanted to come home but Mom said she wanted me to stay in London; she knew I would be coming home to see her and that otherwise I would have wanted to be in London and celebrate with my friends. My birthday fell on a Friday, so she planned to come visit with me and the rest of the gang. I was living in a house with a gas fireplace as the main source of heat—it wasn't ideal for my mom, who was cold all the time now that she had no hair on her head. Getting out of the house was the only logical solution. It was no surprise that we ended up at the mall, because my mom decided that I needed a new shirt to wear out that night. Even though she felt terribly unwell, she insisted on sitting in the change room while we picked out the perfect birthday shirt.

Later we went for dinner and then returned to my house for the dessert that she had brought. I sat on the couch as the lights were turned out and my mom came in with my favourite white Loblaws cake, decorated with a picture of me when I was about five years old. I closed my eyes, made my wish and blew out the candles. As the lights went on, my mom leaned over to me and whispered in my ear, "I will be." She knew what I had wished for and we both started to cry. Shortly after, my "entourage" left and I went directly to my room. I sat on my bed and cried. I called my mom while they were still en route to Toronto, and it was no surprise to her that I was feeling this way. It had been just a matter of time before I broke down.

Before I knew it, Christmas break had arrived. I was not, as one might have expected, going home to spend time with my mom. There had been an ongoing struggle at my family's house about the planned December vacation to Aruba. My dad, sister, brother and I had decided that we would all stay home and that would be the end of it. But even though the score was 4 to 1, the woman of the house overruled us all and sent us on our way while she stayed home to continue with chemotherapy. I was very unhappy about this, but for those of you who don't personally know my mom, let me inform you that you can fight to the death with her, but you will never, ever win. I was relieved to hear that Aunty Zozzie, my mom's sister, who lives in Baltimore, Maryland, would be coming to Toronto to spend the time with her. The vacation was quite different from our usual vacations, to say the least, and we talked to my mom by phone all the time.

January was the end of chemo. The morning it was over I called her, but by the sound of her voice I could tell she wasn't as excited as I thought she would be. She had received many calls congratulating her for finishing chemo, but she didn't see it as a cause for celebration. She saw it only as the end of one step, with many more to go. She still had to have the double mastectomy and the hysterectomy, not to mention the breast expanders and then the implant surgery. She did not see it as over.

The double mastectomy took place over my reading week, so I was able to be at home. The surgery was performed on a Tuesday and by Friday night she was back in her own bed. My mom had been reluctant to take painkillers, but while still in the hospital after this major surgery, she had had enough. She asked the nurse for something to dull the pain. The nurse gave her two pills and told her she might need only one. But both pills were down before the nurse finished her sentence. Very quickly, my mom began to hallucinate. My Aunty Sandy and I were in the room with her and she began talking to herself about some jacket that was "hideous" and she couldn't believe that "she" was wearing it. This was one of the humorous moments. What happened later, however, wiped out that comical memory for a time.

When she came home, I had to learn how to empty the drains that went from the inside of her chest to hang down by her sides. Being squeamish, I found this more difficult than my sister might have, but Amanda had gone with a friend to Collingwood for the weekend (she taught skiing there, and my mother had insisted she go away and celebrate her birthday). Things seemed to be fine, but then suddenly there was hemorrhaging from one of the drain sites. It all happened really fast. I had to make sure that Matt stayed away from her bathroom. I called Vivien Brown right away—she had already been visiting earlier—and asked her to come over as soon as she could. My Aunty Wendy was there, as well as a few of my mom's other friends, and my mom was the calmest of us all as she explained what to do, where to put pressure and how to clean her up. Soon Vivien was there and we all let the doctor take over, but still it was clear that my mom would have to return to the hospital. Wendy offered to drive, but my mom was prepared to stay home rather than get into her low-slung sports car again. I wanted to take her but someone had to stay home with Matt, without letting him know what was going on. Before I knew it they were gone.

I called my dad to tell him to get to the hospital as soon as he could, and then the house was silent. I was in total shock.

It had all happened so fast that there had been no time to be scared. Now it seemed there was time for nothing else. I told Matt that I was going to take a shower. First, though, I wanted to talk to someone. My friends were all over the world, literally. Cheri was still in Israel and I had friends in Australia and British Columbia. Most of my other friends were out of town for reading week. I called a friend in Toronto but she was out; I left a rambling, almost senseless message on her answering machine. I hung up, got into the shower and just cried. I felt completely useless, knowing that my mom was on the way to the hospital and I wasn't with her. I stayed in the shower for as long as I could, until there was no sign that I had been crying. Matt and I went to Wendy's for dinner, and when we got home, Mom was back in bed—just as Matt had last seen her.

A day or two later, my mom felt it was necessary to put on a sports bra that was almost skin-tight. I wasn't there when she put it on, but I was definitely there when she had to take it off. If I had been around when she was getting dressed this would never have happened. Because it was so tight, the only way to get it off was for her to put her arms up over her head, which was basically impossible after a double mastectomy. I wanted to cut it off, but there was no way she was going to let me do that—as far as she was concerned, that was more of an impossibility than getting it over her head. About 40 minutes later we managed to get the sports bra off with only minimal pain. A piece of advice, if I may: there should be no fashion show in your bedroom after surgery of this kind; stay in baggy clothes and zip-up shirts.

Some days were better than others. As the stubborn woman that she is, my mom has always been reluctant to take pain-killers. When she was on them it was better than not. I spent the majority of the week in bed with her. I slept with her every night so that she wouldn't be disturbed when my dad went to work in the morning. The nights and the mornings were the hardest. She rarely slept through the whole night because she could only sleep on her back. She tossed and turned and there was very little I could do but lie awake with her and hope that she would get some sleep. In the mornings I would get her tea and try to get as much food into her as I could, but it was difficult. Within a week or so, she was downstairs eating dinner with us and moving around the house again. That was always what I looked forward to, even while I worried that she gave herself too little time to recuperate. Whenever she went through a surgery or was feeling sick from the chemotherapy, I had to keep in the back of my mind that soon enough she would be downstairs and taking on more than she should. As hard as it was for me to see her in those states, she wanted to be there even less, and I always knew that she would be back on her feet soon enough.

The next big steps were the hysterectomy, which took place in April, and then the final implant surgery in July. Around this time we were able to see some hair growing back on my mom's head. As the days went on, the growth became more and more visible. If there is one thing I know, it is that hair growth in our family is no issue!

On the morning of the breast implant surgery, I went to work, then to the hospital right after. My mom was groggy and clearly in pain. She had to go to the bathroom at one point and asked me to help her up. When she came out of the bathroom she was trembling and unable to stop. Her lips had begun to turn a bluish purple and we were both scared. I called a nurse, who helped me get her back into bed and warm her up. It happened once more that evening, and was probably some sort of reaction to a medication. I had trouble holding back the tears when this would happen, but I did my best. When it was time for me to leave, around 11 p.m., she insisted that I not walk to the underground parking lot alone, so I had some friends meet me in the lobby and we drove home together. All in all it was a very stressful and scary night. I had been alone and no one understood how it had felt. As I was driving home, Cheri called to see how I was, since she knew the surgery had happened earlier that day. When she asked me how I felt I just began to cry. I was crying so hard that I soon pulled over and let someone else take the wheel. I calmed down as I spoke to Cheri but still I cried the entire way home. As we reached home, I said goodbye to Cheri, then apologized to the others in the car with me. They said not to worry about it, but I wished that I hadn't cried in front of them and made them feel uncomfortable.

When my mom came home a day or two later, she had tons of visitors, as usual. This time, though, the atmosphere in her room was different; everyone knew this was the last major surgery and that it marked the end of the long year that we had all faced with her. It must have seemed an entire lifetime to her.

We spent the rest of the summer together since my mom was still unable to go back to work. We went to cottages with friends, met for lunch and shopped, taking advantage of the time we had together. We talked, made plans and actually followed through with them. Unlike the year before, she was able to help me move back to London for school. This adventure to London was a healthy one, with the house warm, my family there with me and my mom feeling energized. It's amazing the difference a year can make.

What seemed like an impossibility just over 12 months ago is now a reality. My mom is healthy, working again, but also home more than she used to be. She has taken off a small load that will benefit both herself and us, her family.

This experience has taught our family so much. There is no law saying that you can experience only so many unfortunate events in one lifetime, but after this experience it is even clearer to me that even bad experiences can be used to benefit someone, somewhere. This isn't the first time that my mom has taken a situation that was detrimental to our family and used it to help others. The Back to Sleep Campaign that my mom was part of made me so proud. I was amazed that she was able to take the death of my brother and talk about it with strangers across Canada. She has been the one who has taught me that we can talk about the bad and turn it into something good, and that is exactly what she did with her battle with breast cancer.

Do I think that my mother's breast cancer will be a lifelong battle for my family? Do I worry that one day it will come back, even after all the precautions she has taken? That is not how I think; it's not the way my mind works. I have been taught throughout my life that we need to live in the present and not in the future. I have learned that I can't live my life thinking about the "what-ifs," because if I do I will forget "what is." And what is right now is that my mom is healthy and she is happy. What is, is that my mom is and always will be the strongest woman I know. What is, is that life is too short and we have to take what we get and be thankful for what we have. To me, our experience with my mother's breast cancer was "what was" and, while it has left a lasting impression on my life, I have to look at what it has brought to my family—which is more strength and love than I ever knew to be possible.

TWENTY-THREE

Amanda's story

It seems like a million years ago my mother sat my sister and me down in our family room to tell us she had been diagnosed with breast cancer. She and my father tried to seem very calm and relaxed about the issue, and my sister had secretly figured it out on her own. So there I sat, shocked, confused and internally not calm or relaxed at all. My first thought was a question: Why was I the only one who had not known? My second thought was that this was not good, not good at all. This was not supposed to happen to my family, not ever—but especially not now! I was about to enter my final year of high school. Wasn't this supposed to be my best year? I had been appointed a prefect at school, which had been a dream of mine since grade 7; I was being given the portfolio I wanted as a prefect; I was supposed to go on a trip to Cancun with all my friends, instruct snowboarding in Collingwood and go on a family vacation to Aruba. This was the year I was going to apply to university, choose where I would go next, wear my white dress to graduation, go to prom and formal and hang out with my friends. My mother having cancer was not part of the plan. This year was supposed to be amazing.

I never imagined that this would happen to my mother and to my family. The only other people I knew personally who had had cancer were my grandfather and the father of one of my best friends. My friend's dad was okay, but we had lost my grandfather to cancer. *We lost my grandfather to cancer*—that was a thought that resonated in my head for a long time after my mother told me about her cancer. My grandfather died because of cancer; was I going to lose my mother to cancer as well? I knew the odds were certainly in my mother's favour, but having to think about any odds determining my mother's fate was enough to worry me. I am a pretty factual person and I am used to relying on intellect. I don't always find comfort in facts, but I know them to be true and honest, so as much as I could I tried to look at my mom's illness from a factual standpoint. However, at the same time I am also a pretty emotional person. I tried as best as I could not to show that I was scared, upset or worried—I figured my mom had enough of her own thoughts to worry about. But it is next to impossible to hide your emotions from the people closest to you, especially when they are suddenly always around.

My mom's having cancer really changed the dynamic of our household. My mother is someone who loves to be busy and on the move. She loves her work and it has always taken up a lot of her time. For most of my life my mom wouldn't be around when I left for school in the morning or when I got home in the afternoon. Sometimes she would even get home after dinner. My dad's schedule was very similar to that because he has to commute just under two hours to work every day. This dynamic never bothered me, though I knew it was different from most of my friends' homes. I never felt like my mom wasn't around enough, and she always made sure to spend her entire weekend with the family. This type of a schedule worked well for me because I like my independence and I like to have my own agenda. It has been a long time since someone has told me to go upstairs and do my homework. I have always had to take responsibility for myself. Doing my work and fulfilling any other commitments I had was always under my charge.

Suddenly, though, my mother was always home. She was there when I left for school in the morning and got home in the afternoon. She was there if I called home in the middle of the day to tell someone I would be home late, and she was there for every dinner. She was always there. In the beginning it was nice, but soon I began to feel a little stifled. It was a big adjustment to always have a parent at home, and my mom was aware that her constant presence took getting used to for everyone. My mom was very good about it. At the time we had someone working for us and I remember watching her try-ing to carry out some sort of task as my mom was watching. It seemed like the most irritating thing. I talked to the woman working for us and asked her if it bothered her; she smiled at me and said, "Of course it bothers me a little, but imagine how your mother feels."

When something bad happens, many people—even ones you don't know—want to show their support for you. They want to be able to help you and reach out to you in any way that they can. They want you to know that you are in their prayers, on their minds and in their hearts. Most of the time, it is a genuine concern for your wellbeing that people are trying to express. At times, however, being on the receiving end of all those warm wishes can be overwhelming. For a long time after my mom went public about her breast cancer, there was a new bunch of flowers, box of candy or small trinket every day. The house smelled like a flower shop! It was incredibly kind, but also a constant reminder that something big was happening, and not in a good way. It was hard at first to get used to all of that.

After the flowers and the letters came the phone calls. The phone would ring constantly for a few hours every day. It got to the point where I would pick up the phone knowing exactly what I would say: "No, I'm sorry, she is busy . . . of course I will tell her you called . . . thank you . . . thank you . . . that's very kind." It must have been so amazing for my mom to feel the support of so many different people, but again it was a constant reminder of something that was wrong in her life. In all of our lives. It got to the point where I had no desire to answer the phone in my house anymore.

It turned out, however, that I didn't need to answer the phone at my house anymore. Why? Well, because shortly after the phone calls came the visitors! It was pretty amazing. From September to November almost every time I came home from school there would be an extra car parked in our driveway. At the beginning it was hard to figure out whose car it could possibly be, but I would make a game out of guessing which car belonged to which of my mom's friends. The visitors—and their cars—settled down to a regular, steady group of my mom's closest friends. By mid-October I had the game down to an art! This group of friends continued to visit all the way through my mom's treatment. They would take my mom down to the hospital for surgeries or chemotherapy, or they would bring her the newest issue of *Vogue, Us* or *People*. My mom was lucky to have such a committed group of friends. They tried to make sure that she was as entertained as possible. For once, my mom was forced to slow down, which may not have been in the end such a bad thing. I think it was probably nice for my mom to have the opportunity to spend so much uninterrupted time with her friends.

For me, personally, it was difficult to always have people around the house, simply because it was such a change from what I was used to. Knowing how much my mom enjoyed the company of her friends, I chose not to complain. I remember one day sitting in my guidance counsellor's office, crying and telling her how all the visitors were driving me crazy. It's not as though they were intruding on my life, telling me what to do or when to do it. But it was still a lot to handle for some reason. My guidance counsellor calmed me down and asked me if I had told my mom. I told her I couldn't. It was not that I felt my mom wouldn't understand, but it was because I wanted her to have the people around her. I felt as though I was being dramatic and I didn't like that feeling. What reason did I have to be upset with any of this? I chose instead to distance myself. I spent a lot of time in my room with the door shut and I would do my work. After a while, my new routine and the quiet of my room began to feel normal.

At school, I was prefect, so I worked closely with the dean of students and the head of the senior and middle school. I remember specifically telling them, on two different occasions, that I really did not want the teachers to approach me about my mother having cancer, and that I just did not want to discuss it at school. They were both incredibly supportive and told me that they would tell the staff not to talk to me about it. The head of the senior and middle school was especially supportive. She let me know that any time I ever needed to get away from everything or if anything was too overwhelming, her door was always open to me. She was so sincere; I could tell she had said those things because she really meant them, not because it was her job. She knew before I did that my mother's cancer was going to affect my life. She was a voice of experience and reason who explained that even though I was not the one with cancer, it was normal for me to feel upset, overwhelmed, scared, alone and any of the million other feelings that I did at some point feel. In retrospect it was really good for me to hear someone say that it was normal to feel a little crazy.

At first I felt like I could keep school and home separate. It turns out that I was wrong. You cannot always set boundaries in your life that block out your emotions. I remember being at school and running into a teacher who is always very bubbly and excited. She used to make us do math aerobics so we could remember the different mathematical functions she was teaching. She has always been a fan of my mom's. The first time they ever met and my teacher realized that my mom was "that woman who hosted *Balance*" she was excited, to say the least. She approached me in the hall and wrapped her arms around me. She told me she was thinking of my family and hoped everything was okay. She said how upsetting the news was to her—to think that someone so healthy could be diagnosed with breast cancer seemed so unfair. As if I didn't already know! Of course she was trying her best to be supportive and just wanted to express her concern for me, but at that point it became clear: there was no separating my mom's breast cancer from the rest of my life.

I put off telling my friends about my mom's breast cancer for as long as possible, but once it was in the newspapers, it was a little hard to avoid the subject. One of my best friends, Julia, knew right from the very beginning. I called her the night my mother told us. I needed her to know. Julia and I became friends at Branksome Hall, our school, but for our final year Julia was going to school in Switzerland. It was one of the points in my life when I needed a best friend the most, and she was getting ready to leave. It made everything just a little bit harder. We e-mailed each other a lot and spoke on the phone when we could, but time-zone differences and busy schedules made it pretty hard. I remember the day that she left I went with her family and her boyfriend to drop her off at the airport, and after I got home I sat in my car and called my sister and cried. My sister was already back at university at this point and I felt pretty alone. My parents knew I was upset about Julia's leaving, so when I was sad the day of her departure they weren't surprised.

Mostly, I tried not to be upset around the house or make my mom worry too much about how I was feeling, although I know that she did anyway. I didn't tell my parents that I had told Julia, but I am sure they knew. With Julia gone my mom was really concerned that I needed to tell someone else. A few days before the public announcement was made, my mom told me that I had to tell someone before I exploded or got too stressed out from it all. That's when I started to tell a few of my other friends. The next to know after Julia was another one of my closest friends, Erin. She came over the night that I told her and hung out with me. We didn't really talk about the cancer too much but having her there was nice. She told me to call her if I ever needed anything or wanted to get out for a little. I've never been one to accept those offers, even from my best friends, but I took her up on it many times! I thought I could deal with everything on my own, but I couldn't. I still can't! I don't think very many people can without feeling like they are going a little insane. Erin lives really close to me and so whenever I didn't feel like being alone I would call her and she would do stuff with me, even boring little things like driving Hebrew school car pool. She was my rock and she made sure that I never crumbled.

After that I told a few more of my closest friends and let everyone else find out as the gossip swirled around the hallways of schools and through the mouths of people, as it usually does. My best friend from camp, Lauren, called me one night and flat out asked me if there was anything I needed to talk about or wanted to tell her. I think that I didn't want to tell people because I didn't want it to be a big deal, I didn't want to admit that it was a part of our lives. At that point it became pretty clear that everyone I knew was going to know. I told her about my mom, and of course she said that she already knew and that she was there for me. She really meant it too. There was a tremendous amount of support from everyone, and I was surprised to find that most of it was genuine.

At Branksome when you are a prefect the school sends you on a leadership retreat weekend so that the prefect group has a chance to become better friends and figure out what leadership styles work best with the specific group dynamics. When I came home from this weekend my head was a little itchy. I couldn't quite figure it out. I decided to go to the health centre at school and check it out. Sadly, I had lice. The nurse called my mom and told her. She proceeded to tell her that I would be asked to leave school for the next 24 hours and that my entire family needed to be checked for lice. The nurse was telling my mom that she would also have to be checked. My mom replied that no, she didn't. The nurse was adamant; my mother had to be checked. My mom answered her in this completely calm voice and said, "I have cancer and my hair is about to fall out, so no, I don't need to be checked." This poor nurse just about fell off her chair! After that, every time I saw her she was incredibly kind and let me know that if I ever needed anything she was around.

The initial shock wore off at school and at home and things got back to normal more or less. Some days were good, some days were worse. Everything was not perfect, but it was okay. I started to like having my mom home more. She would get bored during the day, so when she was feeling up to moving around she would make her own soups and bake really good cookies and cakes. That part was really nice. Other parts, however, were not as nice! Early in the process, for instance, my mom had stitches in her breasts and somehow they came undone and she started to bleed. It was a weekend and my dad and brother were out. My sister was already at university and I was the only one home with my mom. She was lying in her bed and all of a sudden I heard her hollering my name. Her bandages were soaked through with blood and she looked a little scared. Together we patched her back up and I called her friend Vivien, who is a doctor, and she came straight over. Everything ended up being fine, but it was really scary for a few minutes. My mom was great through it all; neither of us freaked out and she calmly told me exactly what I needed to do. I can't imagine that the situation would have been handled as calmly if she hadn't been able to doctor herself. I had never imagined trying to patch my mother's nipple back onto her breast—but then again, what daughter has?

Every year, midway through October, Branksome holds a ceremony called the Installation of the Prefects. It is a big ceremony, held in a church, in which all the school's leaders are inducted into their positions. Because I was a prefect in my graduating year, the ceremony meant a lot to me. I had been attending the ceremony for the previous five years hoping one day I would be among the inductees. Needless to say, the morning of the ceremony I was eager to get moving, but when I walked into my parents' room my dad pulled me aside and told me that my mom wasn't feeling so good and that she probably wasn't going to be able to come. I immediately tried to hide my disappointment and pretended that it didn't bother me. I know she saw right through me. She told me she was sorry and I didn't have much to say. It wasn't that I was upset with her, it was that this ceremony was something special to me and I had wanted so badly to share it with her. I wanted her to sit in a pew at that church and see me and be proud.

I had to be at the church a few hours early for pictures and then we were taken into the basement to wait for the ceremony to start. It was only once they called my name to stand before the audience that I saw my mom sitting with my dad, with tears streaming down her face. I was shocked. It was such a good feeling to know that she was watching me. It was an even better feeling to know that although she had been feeling so sick she could still manage to be there if she tried really hard. That was a good day.

In December my family usually goes away for the Christmas break. That year we were supposed to go to Aruba. My sister, my dad and I were feeling a little unsure about going because that meant we would have to leave my mom at home. My mom, however, was not unsure; she absolutely wanted us out of the house. Her sister was coming to stay with her and she didn't want us hanging around making a mess for a week and making her life more stressful. So, come December, we went to Aruba and left my mom at home for a week. It was difficult and I felt guilty about it. I know she was happy to have her sister there but it didn't feel right going away without her. The vacation felt weird, and a lot of the nights my sister and I would just go back to the room with my brother, Matt, who was nine at the time. We let my dad stay out most nights with the adults, although I know he didn't stay out very long. Everything on the vacation was beautiful and wonderful, but it just felt really strange without my mom.

However, I did get the chance to go away with just my mom a little after the December holidays. My mom and I went to Palm Beach in Florida as an early birthday present for me. I was happy to spend some time, just me and her. We stayed at a beautiful hotel and it was in a nice quiet area. At this point my mom was done with all of her chemotherapy. Her hair was just starting to grow back: she had a little peach fuzz and it was incredibly exciting! We went to Florida because my mom's immune system was not incredibly strong and she wasn't supposed to leave North America. At this point it was definitely a bad idea for her to be exposed to sickness of any kind, including a cold. On the last night of the trip I got sick. I was puking in the bathroom, and at first I was nervous that I had gotten some bug that my mom might catch, but luckily it turned out to be only food poisoning.

Throughout the months of January and February things progressed with my mother's treatment. On February 15, the day before my birthday, my mom was undergoing some serious surgery. We would only be able to see my mom on the 16th, my birthday. I was a racer on the Branksome snowboarding team, and had been for four years. My final race was on February 16. The team had been training all semester and this was my last competition as a member of it. Going to the race meant I wasn't going to be back in Toronto until late at night, and I wanted to be able to go to the hospital as soon as possible after my mom's surgery. I chose not to go to the race, but didn't tell my parents. I could have gone and it would have been fine, but I would have been worried all day. I wouldn't have been able to perform well. My mom felt badly that her surgery was so close to my birthday. She apologized a lot but I was okay with it. My dad gave me tickets to a Toronto Raptors game and told me that after I saw my mom I should go to the game and try to enjoy my birthday. I went down to the hospital to see my mom. She looked pretty wrecked. I didn't feel good seeing her like that, but I kept telling myself that this was the only way she could get better. As soon as she saw me she tried to be as bright as possible and wished me a happy birthday. I'm not sure if that made me feel better or worse about everything.

After I went to the hospital I went home. Jenna surprised me for my birthday and came home from university. We went to the basketball game and about halfway through the game my name came up in lights on the Jumbotron—it was a birthday wish that my mom and dad had arranged for me. The Raptors Dance Pack came out and did a whole birthday dance. It was exceedingly embarrassing, but I loved it and I can't begin to describe how hard Jenna and I laughed. Being with my sister at a basketball game and just laughing made me forget for a little while about everything else. So I guess even that was a good day.

Oftentimes you need to escape for a little, and laughing has always been a good way for me to do that. I don't see myself as particularly funny, but I think my friends are. We laughed a lot last year, and it was good, especially for me. We tried to laugh as much as we could at home too. Of course things are serious, but if there is no laughter at all, not only are things serious but they are scary! Both my parents were always very open about all the treatment that my mom had to go through. Although they were being honest with us and telling us serious information, they tried to joke sometimes about what was going on. My mom was telling me once about a meeting with one of her surgeons about the reconstructive phase and she was telling me that my dad had asked if he got to choose the new size. As much as I try not to think about what my parents do when we aren't around, it was good to know that they were bringing a little humour into the experience.

My dad is an amazing guy. He was always smiling and joking around, trying to keep everyone happy. He's good at it! Every winter my family goes skiing in Collingwood on the weekends. Last year it was just my dad, my brother and me. Driving to Collingwood takes about two hours. I would drive, Matt would sleep and my dad would take out his iPod and we would play music games. We would play all the songs that started with the word "love" or all the songs that started with a girl's name. Having those two hours together in the car every Friday and Sunday made it easy for me to talk to my dad about anything that was on my mind. I had never had the opportunity to spend so much time with just my dad, and though of course I had always been able to talk to him when I wanted, or call him whenever, this was different. He would ask about school and all the things in my life, and instead of just saying everything was fine I started to tell him if I was fighting with a friend or who I was taking to formal. He was a good listener and sometimes had some good advice.

Those weekends in Collingwood felt pretty normal, even without my mom. My mom would pack us a big food bag before we left the house, so that was always taken care of! My dad assumed a little bit of a different role than he had before; he would refill the lunch pack, make the dinner plans, save seats at the table for us and get whatever groceries we needed. At first it was weird, because my dad had never done those things, my mom always had! By the end of the season the weekends with my dad were as coordinated and as organized as the ones with my mom. It felt like nothing was really different.

During March break almost all the private-school students in grade 12 go away to Cancun, Mexico, together. I had been hearing about this trip since I was in grade 7 at Branksome—it was a tradition. Luckily for me, I got to go too. My parents knew that it was something I had always really wanted to do and there was almost no discussion of my not going. It was weird to leave my mom again for another week, but it was different from our December holiday because there were no reminders of the fact that my mom wasn't there—no one's mom was there.

That week in Cancun was a really good mental break for me. I forgot about everything at home and had fun with my friends. There was no use in being there if I was going to be miserable! Just because my mom was sick, though, didn't mean that she stopped parenting me. Oh no! She sat me down on numerous occasions to have the "safe travelling without the parents" talk. No walking alone, eating alone, going to the beach alone or doing anything alone. No taking drinks from strangers, no leaving drinks unattended or talking with strangers. No drugs and no stealing. Of course a lot of this would never apply to me and my mother knew that, but she still repeated it 152 times! My mother may have been sick, but she was still my mother.

My mom cut her hair really short because she knew it was going to fall out sooner or later. She had two wigs and she named them; one was Judy and the other was Janice. I recall one day my mother saying to my brother, "Matt, can you go please take Judy out of the box? She'll suffocate otherwise." At this point my brother wasn't aware of the naming of the wigs. The look on his face was priceless. My mom picked up on his clueless air immediately and explained. He may have been shocked and creeped out, but my sister and I thought it was hilarious.

Bandanas and headbands were never really an option for my mom. She wore either a lululemon cap or a fleece cap, or occasionally a baseball cap if she was going out. She had this one little orange fleece hat that she slept with because her head would get cold. Every time she put it on she told us she felt like one of the seven dwarfs. It was very cute! People used to buy my mom silly gifts, including a big silly straw hat with the Burberry pattern on it. Jenna and I thought it was a very funny hat, so one late spring day we took it from the house, along with another silly hat, a fur one, and went grocery shopping and for coffee in them. People stared at us, and I am sure they were wondering what on earth we were doing. I keep the picture of my sister wearing that silly hat right beside my bed, to remind me of that day and to remind me that everything turned out pretty amazingly.

Matt and I became very close last year. He and I were the only kids in the house, so we spent a lot of time together. When I got home from school he would come to my room and lie down on the floor to do his homework while I did mine. He would always tell me everything about his day and make me laugh one way or another. Because I could drive, I would sometimes drive the Hebrew school car pool and he would make up silly excuses for not going. He would say things that I used to tell my mom when I didn't want to go to Hebrew school, so I would just laugh. It was funny because I knew all the tricks and he still tried them anyway. I would also take Matt to his soccer and hockey games and he would tell me about the really bossy kid on the team or how he was going to score so much. I have always worried about the big age gap between Matt and me and Matt and Jenna. I've worried that he won't feel like I can understand him and be his friend because I am so much older. Now I worry a little less. Right now I am away at school and Matt is the only one at home, but because we got to be so close to each other last year he does trust me. He knows that even though we are so far apart in age I think that everything he has to say is important.

Matt and I go to the same summer camp. I am a staff member and he is a camper. During the summer my mom had one of her surgeries and the plan was that my mom would call the camp afterwards and we would be able to talk to her. Matt came to my cabin before we had to be at the office so that we could walk there together. He looked at me and gave me a big hug and grabbed my hand. We went to the office and spoke to my mom, who actually sounded very good, though a little tired, and then I started to walk him back to his cabin. Halfway there I sat him down on the steps of the health centre and I asked him if he was okay or if he was worried. He said no and that he was just happy he got to talk to her. He gave me another hug and then ran the rest of the way back to his cabin.

My sister has always been a really good friend to me, but last year she was especially great. We get along well because we balance each other out. Jenna used to wish that she could be at home with the family and I would sometimes wish that I could go away. Seeing my mom sick was so hard for me. My mother has never been one to sit still for longer than 15 minutes, so it was difficult to see her restricted to the house at times and sometimes even to her bed. Jenna and I are really close. We have completely different academic interests, but other than that we are extremely similar. Whenever I was feeling a little sad or scared I would call Jenna up and she could take my mind off it or make me feel better about it really fast; when she was sad I could do the same for her. Jenna came home from school as many times as she could to show her support for my mom, but her coming home also helped me a lot. I love having Jenna around the house; she always makes it feel a little more alive.

I guess you could say I am pretty lucky. My mother is a trooper and a fighter. During every chemotherapy treatment, during every surgery and every type of test that she was put through, she stayed positive. Sure, at times that positive energy ran a little lower than others, but underneath it was always there. You have to believe that things are going to be okay, because if you lose hope, imagine how easy it would be for everyone around you to give up hope, to give up their battle. I learned a lot about myself and my family through my mom's fight with breast cancer. I learned a lot about what is truly important in this life, and about how to live it.

Ever since I was little my parents told me that I had to live life to the fullest. Before my grandfather died he told my dad that he had lived his life to the fullest, that he had no regrets and that he was happy. Throughout everything my mom was going through she always told me she had no regrets. She has done everything that she has wanted to do. She leads this amazing life, with a huge family who loves her and great friends. I think her battle helped my whole family step back and re-evaluate how we live our lives. I feel that my mom's priorities have changed, and mine as well. My mom has slowed down the pace of her life a little, which I think is good for her. The rest of us, well, we were reminded just how important our family and friends are to us. We learned a lot about making sure that what is really important in our lives—like each other—gets enough attention. So maybe my year hadn't been the amazing one that I'd planned for, but it was amazing in an entirely different way. It was a learning experience. When you think about it, if you can't rely on your family, whatever family that may be, who can you trust to catch you when you fall or pick you up when you're stumbling?

TWENTY-FOUR

Matt's story

Hi. I'm Matthew, the youngest one in the family. When I first found out my mom had breast cancer I was very shocked because my mom is a doctor. She is always healthy. When I understood that it was true and not a dream—I wasn't imagining, she actually had cancer—I was scared . . . but I was hoping. First I was hoping it wasn't true, then I was hoping she would just get better. Everyone said she was a fighter and I believe them . . . . She is.

I found out she had cancer because something happened that never happens—a family meeting. My sisters knew about the cancer, but I didn't. Jenna, who is my oldest sister, wrote an e-mail to my mom saying, "You are a fighter, you are going to beat it." I saw her writing it not long before the family meeting and I got scared. So I sort of had an idea that my mom must be very sick. The meeting was right after dinner, and Mom told us what was going on. I started asking questions, like "Why will you lose your hair?" and "Why is there more than one surgery?" She tried to explain everything to me.

One day all of her hair was gone, and when I first saw her I said, "Don't take off your hat, you will look scary." She went to her room and she was just sad from then on. I got used to her being bald because as time went on I knew things would be okay, so I just called it a side effect, nothing more than a side effect. To me it meant that the treatment must be working.

When my friends saw her they were all surprised and asked what happened. I told them the truth, saying she had breast cancer. Most of my friends said oh, and they were scared. The others asked if she was going to be okay. I told them that I didn't know, but I hoped she would be.

People stared at my mom when she went out bald. I was used to her by that time and it just was normal. Some people talked about her and some thought she cut her hair. But she had NO hair. It was gone, not like when I get a really short buzz. Sometimes people would just stare and stare. Maybe it was because they knew who she was. Once I turned around and said, "Don't worry—it's going to grow back."

My mom had to take these needles at home. I hate needles. I hate when my mom brings me home a flu shot and wants to give me a needle. I thought it was weird that my mom had to give herself needles every day, but I kind of understood that she could do it. She is a doctor and knows how. She would sometimes forget to do it in the morning. I would count the days with a chart I made, and every day I would ask her if she took her needle.

On the day of her very last needle, I made a big sign. It was an important day. I stuck the sign on the fridge. It said, Congratulations on your last nidil. You are done. My mom of course taught me how to spell it right!

When my mom was in her treatment she was home a lot. It was fun for me because when I got home from school it wasn't just me and my babysitter. She was always there. She always wanted to know if I wanted to bake cookies with her. I said yes. I got good at baking chocolate chip cookies. I have always been good at eating them, but now I know how to make them too. We also made Smarties cookies, macadamia nut cookies, fudge brownies and my all time favourite, ooey gooeys. Those are chocolate brownies with marshmallows on top and lots of chocolate sauce. My mom doesn't eat them. I am the only one. But she does bake them.

In the summer I left to camp, and that day my mom had a big surgery. So I called home just to see if she was okay. She was. She was talking very weakly and she sounded very tired. I went back to my cabin happy, very happy. My two best friends were there and they already knew. So they didn't ask anything because they thought they had to keep it a secret. It wasn't, maybe to them but not to me. When I saw my mom on visitors' day she had a lot of hair. I really couldn't believe it. It was short and curly. She wasn't bald anymore. Now today my mom is perfectly fine, with a full head of hair.

I think my mom's cancer is gone. It will never come back. She hasn't told me that, but I know that every morning she takes a pill. Its name is Arimidex, and I know that because she keeps it in her bathroom. I know what is happening. She doesn't hide things from me. She says it's important to take the pill to keep the cancer away. She does tell me there are no guarantees, like it's not for sure that it won't come back. I say it's not for sure it will come back. So I am right. It won't.

My mom is back to her crazy schedule. It's really good that she is back. It feels normal, just like it did before she got her cancer. It really is good.

At the beginning it felt really scary but towards the end, you just know what is going to happen. You can't say someone is going to live because you don't know, but you can't say they are going to die either. So my advice is not to think about it. Life feels more normal that way. It feels better.

TWENTY-FIVE

Bobby's story

My phone rang and it was Susan. I knew it was not good news if Susan was calling. In my 25 years with Marla there have been very few times when she could not speak.

My stomach was in a knot as Susan told me that the results were not good. Finally, she put Marla on the phone. There are defining moments in every life and this was one in mine. Hearing the fear in Marla's voice really scared me. She doesn't scare easily. She had given bad news to many patients over the years, but this was about her. She started telling me the details, the timeline of what lay ahead. But I was in shock. How could this be happening? *Marla is the healthiest person I know. She eats right, exercises, does all the right things. It must be a mistake.* So many thoughts were going through my head: Marla, the kids, our parents, our brothers and sisters. Everything changed that day.

Later, when I got home, we hugged and I tried to reassure her. I knew it wasn't working. Maybe I was trying to reassure myself.

From one doctor's appointment to another we waited for results until a definitive diagnosis was made. The cancer's type, size and location were analyzed and a course of action was decided. Though in retrospect it seemed to go very fast, at the time the process felt excruciatingly slow. Marla and the doctors had the next approximately 12 months planned, procedure by procedure. It was to be a long road, with many difficult decisions to make along the way, no "right" answers and not a lot of time to think. Chemo, radiation, mastectomy, or not? These were decisions that required a lot of soul-searching about what our future would hold. We tried to keep our lives as normal as possible with this huge cloud over our heads.

As a couple, Marla and I have always been open with our kids. This was going to be no different, but it would be very difficult. We have had to deal with a few more tragedies than most families. The loss of our son 13 years ago took its toll on all of us. Telling our daughters was a very difficult moment. You could see the fear in their eyes, while Marla was trying to be upbeat. They had so many questions and we didn't have the answers. That uncertainty made it especially hard to do what every parent wants to do—protect your kids from all the bad things in this world. Throughout all of this, uncertainty was one of the hardest things. We were always wondering what would come next, which way the road would take us and how we would adjust to each situation.

But Marla is an unbelievable person—driven, caring, compassionate and loving. She has enormous strength, and when she sets her mind to something there is no stopping her. She wasn't going to let cancer stop her. She made sure to keep herself busy and to find ways to contribute. She accepted an assignment to write biweekly for the *Globe and Mail* and continued to do *Canada AM* no matter how sick she felt. She knew herself well enough to realize that she needed these things to give her a purpose and a reason to get up in the morning. It allowed her to put the cancer aside, if only for a few moments. It helped her to forget.

I think the hardest thing for Marla through the year-long battle was to let people in, to let her guard down and be vulnerable. She is a fantastic friend who always puts others first, always wants to make things easy for others. She found it hard to let go. It took a while but she finally did and allowed all of us—her family and mine, our children and our amazing group of friends—to help her. Friends and family members took Marla to appointments, visited regularly, drove carpools, cooked meals and took her out when she felt well enough. One even gave her foot massages. The e-mails and phone calls were sometimes overwhelming, but our friends and family were tremendously supportive and would do anything for us, and we couldn't have come through this without them.

Watching my partner slowly deteriorate physically was just a horrible, horrible ordeal. Marla had eight sessions of chemo, each of which completely drained her physical energy for a time. The surgeries and recoveries, being in and out of hospitals, the pain, the pills—it was an emotional nightmare to watch Marla go through so much. I was fortunate, though, that during this period of time my business was stable, and my very good staff made it possible for me to take as much time as I needed to be with Marla. Not everyone in my situation has that luxury.

I am also very lucky to have many good friends in whom I was able to confide on the bad days. I needed people to talk to, to let out my fears and frustrations. You don't need them to give you advice but you do need them to listen. It really helped. During the time that Marla was undergoing chemo, one of my oldest childhood friends took ill in Montreal. Week by week before Christmas 2004 he kept deteriorating. We had gone to summer camp together many times, beginning when we were 10 years old, and we spent so much time with each other's family as we grew up that we became like family to one another. We had spoken almost every week for the past 25 years. Lawrence was a true friend who was always there for me when I needed him and I know he felt the same about me. Lawrence passed away December 24, 2004. He is sorely missed by his family and friends. I will never forget him.

Marla's decision to go public in breast cancer awareness month was hugely courageous. There would be no secrets; everyone would know. Breast cancer affects one out of every nine women in North America. Going public could only help the awareness, and the fundraising. If breast cancer could happen to Marla, it could happen to anyone.

Marla also decided early on to document her experience and started writing this book from the beginning. I know it really helped her emotionally to put her feelings down in print. She also pitched the idea of the documentary, *Run Your Own Race,* to CTV early on. The end result was a very moving and informative hour about all the ups and downs that we had gone through, that other patients also go through. In many ways it demystified all the tests, procedures, surgeries and decisions that women must go through when they are fighting breast cancer. But it was a very emotional process for Marla as she re-lived the previous year, the doctors' diagnoses and action plans, along with their fears. My daughters' and my small interviews just helped to show that any illness affects not only the patient but the whole family. There really isn't a lot of attention given to the families of cancer patients.

Our children are amazing—smart, loving, caring and so devoted to each other. My girls, having lost their brother Jason when they were quite young, have been through more grief than most adults. Losing him left them with some emotional scars, though Marla and I have tried very hard to help them heal. Cancer was their latest battle to fight. Jenna's being away, coming home on weekends to be with her mother and then going back, was terribly stressful for her. Amanda, in her graduating year of high school, was home and living it every day while keeping up with her studies—it was more than a young person should have to deal with. Matthew, just a little boy, saw his mother ill every day and wondered what would happen. We tried to keep things as normal as possible, but there were times when it was very hard. The girls love their brother so much. Now that they are both away at school they still try to talk to him every day. They can't wait to do things with him when they come home. I truly believe they are each other's best friends and can tell each other everything. We are so proud of all three of them. They are very special.

This past year has brought us all closer together. We have always been close but the fear of losing someone you love puts everything in perspective. Marla is well now and back to her busy self, but with some changes. We are stronger as a couple, and as a family. She has put more balance in her life, knowing how fragile it can be. She is more committed than ever to helping people and to helping herself. What is important has a different meaning now. Everything can change in an instant. We cannot change the past. We have no crystal ball to predict our future. We can only live for today.

Acknowledgements

I could not have written this book without the support, encouragement and endless patience of my family. To Bobby, who knows who I really am and told me to ask not *if*, but *when*, and to Jenna, Amanda and Matt—you are the teachers who taught me how to find my own personal balance.

I am enormously lucky to be surrounded by a family that is always there for me. To my parents, Sylvia and Max, mother-in-law Julie, Zozzie, David, Wendy, Alan, Sandy and Eddie—I can never tell you how much your care and love sustained me through the most difficult of times.

I am fortunate to have what I fondly call a board of directors populated by amazing friends, friends who do not understand the words "no" or "go away," friends who constantly transported me to happier places and times, and kept reminding me to believe that another day would come. Susan, Renee and Anne, along with all my other pillars—you touch me every day and remind me how truly lucky I am.

Thanks to my colleagues at *Canada AM* and CTV, to Jordan and Wendy—you allowed me to retain my integrity and identity when I needed them most. To Barb and my office staff, you gave me peace of mind every day, reminding me it was just a matter of time until I could come back to everything I so desperately missed.

Special thanks to my literary agent, Rick Broadhead, who believed I could write a book years ago, long before I ever considered writing a column, much less a book. Thanks to Sylvia Stead of the *Globe and Mail,* and my *Globe* health editor, Kathryn Maloney, who patiently worked with me in sculpting my health columns. To Jim Gifford, Miranda Snyder and all the people at HarperCollins who have been behind me since day one, I thank you. Thank you to David Kent and Iris Tupholme for your enthusiasm, and Phyllis Bruce for your unwavering support of my book from the beginning. And most important, to Nicole Langlois, my amazing editor, who nursed me through the painful edits and went head-to-head with me whenever I dug my heels in—you just dug yours in a little harder.

To all my doctors and caregivers, David McCready, Karina Bukhanov, Joan Lipa, Joan Murphy, Maureen Trudeau and Susan Love, as well as my special friend Vivien, all of whom had the onerous task of supporting me, educating me and treating me—"thank you" falls well short of how I feel. Thanks to Stacy, who kept me strong physically and has included her training program in this book. Thank you to Bonnie Stern for being the amazing support she was and for allowing me to include her recipes in my book. As well, a smile and a chuckle to Robert Buckman who, along with his e-hugs, has written his thoughts on humour and healing in this book.

And finally, I thank my patients and all the men and women who wrote, e-mailed and prayed for me. This is a journey that should never be taken alone. When we are confronted with such a journey, we must draw strength from each other. Courage finds you and, in turn, you find courage.

Bonnie Stern's feel-better comfort food

Although Marla and I didn't know each other well, our paths had crossed in many ways. My son Mark worked on her television show as a production assistant, and one of my best friends, Randy Gulliver, was the first director on her show. Our daughters attend the same university, and Marla even took cooking classes from me when she first moved to Toronto. When I heard she had breast cancer, I knew she had a large network of close friends and that she wouldn't need me to do things like sit with her at the hospital. I thought about what I could do that others might not, and so I offered to cook. I did not commit to making all her meals as it was a busy time at my cooking school (don't make promises you can't keep!) but said I would adapt some of my recipes according to what she could tolerate, and if she liked something in particular I would tell her how to make it. I would randomly send meals over by cab (I didn't want her to feel she had to entertain me if I brought the food in person), and her heartfelt emails made me wish I could help more. You never know what something means to someone when you reach out.

Some hints about cooking for someone who is sick:

- Resist the urge to start cooking without first asking about food preferences and restrictions. You are cooking for your friend, not yourself, and you want to be sure you cook the right things. Remember that people with compromised immune systems may need to avoid certain foods.
- Do not worry that you are just using a few ingredients or that the recipes are very simple.
- Stay away from spices unless you ask about each one specifically.
- Stay away from acidic ingredients like lemon juice, vinegar and tomatoes.
- Stay away from garlic, onions, hot peppers, red peppers and other ingredients that are hard to digest.
- "Comfort" foods are often welcomed.
- Keep flavours gentle.
- Offer your friend a list of recipes to choose from.

Good luck!
—Bonnie Stern

The recipes found on the following pages are © Bonnie Stern Cooking Schools Ltd., reprinted with permission.

Egg White and Spinach Frittata

You can use 8 whole eggs or 16 whites or anything in between, as long as you have 16 parts in all. For example, if you want to use half whole eggs and half whites, you will need 4 whole eggs (2 parts each), and 8 whites.

6 oz (175 g) baby spinach

16 egg whites

8 oz (250 g) bocconcini (fresh buffalo mozzarella) or mild feta
   cheese, drained and broken into bits (optional)

Pinch of salt

Pinch of grated nutmeg

1. Place spinach in a large glass bowl and microwave 30 to 60 seconds or until just wilted. Do not add any liquid. (Or cook in a deep skillet over medium heat, turning spinach with tongs, for 1 to 3 minutes or until just wilted.) When spinach is cool enough to handle, gently squeeze out excess liquid.

2. Place egg whites and spinach in a food processor and pulse until spinach is chopped and mixture is foamy. Add cheese if using, salt and nutmeg. Pulse briefly to mix.

3. Spray an 8-inch (2 L) baking dish with nonstick spray or brush with butter or oil. Pour in egg white mixture. Bake in a 350°F (180°C) oven for 25 to 30 minutes or until set.

Roasted Cauliflower Soup

To keep this soup very gentle, I didn't use any garlic or onions.

1 cauliflower (about 1 ½ lb/750 g), trimmed and broken into
   florets
2 tbsp (25 mL) olive oil
1 tbsp (15 mL) fresh thyme leaves
2 tsp (10 mL) salt
3 cups (750 mL) vegetable or chicken stock or water
1 cup (250 mL) milk (optional)

1. Toss cauliflower with oil, thyme and 1 tsp (5 mL) of the salt.
   Spread in one layer on a baking sheet lined with parchment
   paper and roast in a 400°F (200°C) oven for 20 to 25 minutes or until tender.
2. Combine cauliflower, stock and remaining 1 tsp (5 mL) salt
   in a large saucepan. Bring to a boil. Reduce heat and sim-
   mer for 15 minutes, or until cauliflower is very tender.
3. Purée soup, in batches if necessary, and return to saucepan.
   Add milk (if using) or additional stock or water to thin soup
   if necessary. Heat thoroughly. Season to taste.

Roasted Squash, Baby Spinach
and Bocconcini Salad

MAKES 6 SERVINGS

The skin on the squash is edible if it is smooth and if the squash is firm. Sweet cherry tomatoes can sometimes be tolerated, and excellent-quality balsamic vinegar (unfortunately expensive!) can sometimes be sweet enough to use.

2 lb (1 kg) butternut squash, halved lengthwise, seeded and cut
   into 8 to 12 wedges
2 cups (500 mL) cherry tomatoes (optional)
1 tbsp (15 mL) olive oil
1 tbsp (15 mL) fresh thyme leaves
½ tsp (2 mL) salt
5 oz (150 g) baby spinach leaves
4 oz (125 g) bocconcini (fresh buffalo mozzarella), drained and
   diced

DRESSING:
2 tbsp (25 mL) best-quality balsamic vinegar (optional)
2 tbsp (25 mL) olive oil
½ tsp (2 mL) salt

1. Arrange squash skin side down on a baking sheet lined with parchment paper. Place cherry tomatoes on another baking sheet lined with parchment. Drizzle or spray squash and tomatoes with olive oil and sprinkle with thyme and salt.

2. Roast squash in a 400°F (200°C) oven for 45 to 50 minutes or until tender and browned. Roast cherry tomatoes 12 to 15 minutes or until skin is just starting to split.
3. Line salad plates with a handful of spinach leaves. Arrange squash, tomatoes and cheese on spinach.
4. Drizzle with balsamic vinegar (if using) and olive oil. Sprinkle with salt.

Wheat Berry and Bocconcini Salad with Dill

MAKES 4 TO 6 SERVINGS

Wheat berries are whole wheat kernels and are available at health food stores, bulk food stores and some supermarkets. They take about 1 to 1 ½ hours to cook, so I always make lots and freeze them in 2-cup (500 mL) or 3-cup (750 mL) freezer bags so I can make this salad quickly on the spur of the moment. You could also use brown rice.

1 cup (250 mL) uncooked wheat berries
8 oz (250 g) bocconcini (fresh buffalo mozzarella), drained and
    cut into small pieces
¼ cup (50 mL) black olives, pitted and halved
2 tbsp (25 mL) pine nuts, toasted
2 tbsp (25 mL) chopped fresh dill
2 tbsp (25 mL) chopped chives
2 tbsp (25 mL) chopped fresh parsley
2 tbsp (25 mL) olive oil, or to taste
½ tsp (2 mL) salt, or to taste
1 tbsp (15 mL) lemon juice (optional)

1. Cook wheat berries in a large pot of boiling water for 1 to 1 ½ hours or until tender. Drain. Rinse with cold water and drain well. You should have approximately 2 ½ cups (625 mL).
2. In a large bowl, combine wheat berries, cheese, olives, pine nuts, dill, chives and parsley.
3. Combine oil, salt and lemon juice (if using). Combine gently with wheat berry mixture. Taste and adjust seasoning if necessary.

Patti's Apple Cobbler

MAKES 8 TO 10 SERVINGS

This cobbler is from my friend Patti. It tastes the way comfort food should—apples and cinnamon bubbling around a biscuit topping.

8 apples (combination of Spy and McIntosh), peeled, cored and thickly sliced
½ cup (125 mL) granulated sugar
1 tbsp (15 mL) ground cinnamon

TOPPING:
1 ½ cups (375 mL) all-purpose flour
¾ cup (175 mL) granulated sugar
¾ cup (175 mL) brown sugar
¾ tsp (4 mL) baking powder
Pinch of salt
2 eggs
½ cup (125 mL) melted butter or vegetable oil

1. Toss apples with sugar and cinnamon in a large bowl. Spread evenly in an oiled 13- by 9-inch (3 L) baking dish.
2. Prepare topping by combining flour, granulated sugar, brown sugar, baking powder and salt. Make a well in the centre. Add eggs and beat lightly. With your fingers, combine eggs with flour mixture until crumbly. Sprinkle mixture over apples. Drizzle with melted butter or oil.
3. Bake in a 350°F (180°C) oven for 45 to 55 minutes or until apples are very tender and juicy and topping is golden brown.

Chocolate Chip Cookies

Don't forget the rest of the family—once in a while.

   1 cup (250 mL) salted butter, at room temperature and cut into
      smaller pieces
   1 ½ cups (375 mL) brown sugar
   ¾ cup (175 mL) granulated sugar
   2 eggs
   2 tsp (10 mL) vanilla
   3 ½ cups (875 mL) all-purpose flour
   2 tsp (10 mL) baking soda
   1 ¼ tsp (6 mL) baking powder
   3 cups (750 mL) chopped milk chocolate or chocolate chips

1. In a stand mixer or with a hand mixer, beat butter and granulated and brown sugars until creamy and smooth and light coloured. Add eggs and vanilla. Beat until combined. Do not worry if the mix appears curdled.
2. In another bowl, stir together the flour, baking soda, baking powder and salt. Add to butter mixture and stir just until combined. Beat in chocolate.
3. Form dough into balls, using about 2 tbsp (25 mL) dough at a time and place on baking sheets lined with parchment paper, leaving about 2 inches (5 cm) between cookies for them to spread. Flatten slightly.
4. Bake in a 350°F (180°C) oven for 11 to 13 minutes or until firm on the outside but still soft inside. Switch racks half way if necessary. Cool on racks.

Staying active during
treatment and recovery
by Dr. Stacy Irvine

During Marla's year fighting breast cancer, she continued to exercise regularly. To some people this will sound inadvisable, or worse. But as a chiropractor and Marla's personal trainer, I was in a position to see the powerful effect that exercise had on Marla as she coped with and recovered from many courses of medication and numerous surgeries.

It may be that you are also undergoing cancer treatments, perhaps chemotherapy or mastectomy, as Marla did. And you may or may not have been following an active exercise program prior to your diagnosis and treatment. Whatever your situation or fitness level, appropriate exercise during treatment can be immensely helpful to your recovery. In these few pages I have outlined what Marla and I did to prepare her for the physical challenges of cancer treatment. Her experience may be of help to you. Of course, as with any exercise program, you should speak to your doctor before undertaking any of the exercises listed in the pages that follow.

From the beginning of her battle with cancer, Marla was emphatic that she wanted to continue to exercise, and she asked for my help in developing a program that she could follow no matter what came up in her treatment. I began to look for research evaluating the effects of exercise on breast cancer and chemotherapy treatments. Unfortunately, at that time most of the research was either anecdotal or case-study based. There were a few good studies that had evaluated exercise, but they mostly reported on how patients felt while exercising, not about what exercises to do or what type of exercise was most beneficial. We were on our own.

Marla and I decided that I would come to her house to help with the workouts. Due to her weakened immune system, it would not have been a good idea to work out in a public gym. We agreed to start as soon as possible.

The day I arrived, Marla had been through her first session of chemotherapy and already she had lost weight and looked exhausted. This was quite a shock for me, since I had not seen her for a few months; my last memory was of the healthy Dr. Marla I was used to training at the gym. We went to her basement and began the workout. Not really knowing what to expect, I started with an easy routine and figured I would watch Marla for cues that she was feeling okay or getting too tired. We did a cardio warm-up on a stationary bike and then proceeded into some step-ups and stair work. As the workout continued, I could see glimpses of the Marla I remembered. Her mood brightened and things seemed almost back to normal. We booked another session for a couple of days later.

The next session started slowly again, with a cardio warm-up, lower body exercises, then abdominals and upper body. As the workout progressed, I could see that Marla was starting to feel better. We finished with PNF (Proprioceptive Neuromuscular Facilitation) stretching and I noticed that her range of motion was greatly decreased compared to the last time I stretched with her. At the next workout Marla informed me that she had felt great following our previous session. Her appetite had been better, and she had had more energy that day. This information encouraged me that we were heading in the right direction.

As the weeks went by, we continued our routine consistently. Marla soon realized that there was a definite pattern to how she would feel following the chemotherapy. The first few days after were manageable for working out, but by about the fifth day, the drugs would make her feel so lethargic and nauseated that workouts were not as helpful. We adapted the schedule accordingly, and again Marla was determined to make this work.

Weeks, then months, passed, and we stuck to the routine, even though Marla faced several additional challenges along the way. The first issue to arise was low hemoglobin levels. This was relevant to her physical training since hemoglobin is a determining factor in the blood's ability to carry oxygen. During exercise the body's oxygen demand increases, and the heart and lungs must work harder to compensate. Marla's heart and lungs were already working hard with her everyday activities; the workouts had to be scaled back a bit to allow for more recovery time.

Our next challenge was preparing for the upcoming surgeries. Marla focused on her upper body training during this time because we both knew that after the mastectomy and other surgeries she would be able to do only limited exercise. It was very important for Marla to be able to sit up on her own following the surgery; she wanted to avoid the pain of being moved by others. With this goal in mind, we worked her abs in as many different ways and with as many repetitions as possible. We even imitated the actual movement she would perform when getting up from the bed after surgery. Every time we worked on her abs, Marla emphasized that she was going to do a sit-up after surgery. I was convinced she could do it—and she did. We also worked hard to prepare Marla's pectoral musculature for the reconstruction surgery, since her surgeon was concerned about the size of those muscles and how much they would need to stretch to accommodate the implants. We added more chest work to strengthen the muscles of the chest wall and spent extra time stretching to lengthen those tissues.

Soon it was time for the first reconstructive surgery. We took a few weeks off while Marla recovered. I knew she was feeling better when she let me know that the loss of movement in her arms was driving her crazy because she was not able to do her usual daily activities. We started again with the workouts and focused mainly on lower body and cardio work. During this time, Marla was experiencing acute pain down her right arm, and she went for a diagnostic ultrasound. She was told that the muscles that anchored the arm to the chest wall had been torn; they had likely been affected by the surgery, and some movement after the surgery had caused them to tear. We spent a few weeks treating this area using modalities and soft tissue treatment, and we were both happy when the pain resolved and we were able to add some more upper body work to her routine.

With the chemotherapy treatments finished, Marla was quickly returning to the very healthy, energetic and determined person I remembered. She had gained some more muscle mass, her hemoglobin levels were back to normal and I could tell her resolve was stronger than ever. Over the next few months of training, I watched her fitness levels surpass her pre-diagnosis fitness capabilities. I was truly amazed at the speedy recovery and the pure physical strength I was witnessing in the gym. At the same time, her work schedule took a very busy turn, filling up with lectures and media appearances, and we were counting down the days until she would return to her medical practice. Now that she is back to her full-time practice, we are once again able to discuss interesting cases, and it is obvious that Marla is more at home in the role of caregiver than patient. She continues to work out as much as her busy schedule will allow.

We have both been excited to see new research published in the area of exercise and breast cancer. Studies are now indicating that regular exercise, performed during and after breast cancer chemotherapy, boosts the activity of infection-fighting T-cells and helps to restore the immune system to its pre-chemotherapy level. Marla and I both believed strongly that she was doing the right thing with her workouts, but it is always great when science supports your beliefs.

The following pages include a listing of the exercises we used during Marla's recovery. I grouped the workouts into three types: easy, medium and hard. We chose Marla's workouts based on where she was in the chemotherapy cycle and how she was feeling on any given day. No matter which workout she was doing, Marla often told me that she loved feeling she had some control over her body again, and what a mental break exercise provided from the rest of the time when she felt overwhelmed by medical procedures and chemotherapy drugs.

The workouts serve as a guide to some exercises that can be done at home with very little equipment. (Once again, be sure to consult with your doctor beforehand to make sure these exercises are appropriate for you.) Doing these workouts will keep your muscles strong during your treatment and ready to work for you when you return to your healthy self. If you are a caregiver for someone who is going through this challenging time, encouragement and possibly companionship during workouts may be helpful. But always do things in moderation. This is not the time to set a goal to break a fitness record or do something strenuous that has not been tried before. Always let your energy level be your guide. The best exercise during this time is sub-maximal, and it should feel good while you are doing it. Take lots of time for rest breaks and water breaks, and don't worry about the number of exercises you complete or how heavy the weights are. The most important thing is that you are taking time to do the workout, getting your circulation going and doing something healthy for your body. Remember that exercise is beneficial as a way to take care of your health and speed up recovery. Rest, nutrition and a positive attitude are equally important.

EASY-DAY WORKOUT

Cardio warm-up (10 min)
Active stretching (5 min)
Dumbbell chest presses (10 lbs X 15 reps)
Bicep curls (10 lbs X 15 reps)
Calf raises (20/leg)
Standing squats (20)
Hip lifts (20)
Tricep extensions (5 lbs X 20 reps)
Abdominal curl-ups (20)
Swimmers (20)
PNF (Proprioceptive Neuromuscular Facilitation) stretching (15 min)

MEDIUM-DAY WORKOUT

Cardio warm-up (15 min)
Active stretching (5 min)
Step-ups (20/leg)
Leg lifts, front (20/leg)
Leg lifts, side (20/leg)
Leg lifts, back (20/leg)
Calf raises (20/leg)
Hip lift (30)
Reverse abdominal lifts (30)
Back extensions (25)
Oblique twists (20/side)
PNF (Proprioceptive Neuromuscular Facilitation) stretching
(10 min)

HARD-DAY WORKOUT

Cardio warm-up (15 min)
Active stretching (5 min)
Step-ups (10 lbs X 20/leg)
Ball squats (20)
Dumbbell chest presses (15 lbs X 20)
Hamstring curls (20)
Dips (20)
Bent-knee push-ups (20)
One-leg hip lifts (20/leg)
Straight leg stretches (30)
Double curl-ups (20/side)
Bird dogs (20)
One-arm row (10 lbs X 20 reps)
PNF (Proprioceptive Neuromuscular Facilitation) stretching
(10 min)

ABDOMINAL CURL-UPS: Performed lying on your back with your knees bent and feet flat on the floor. Slowly curl up to a sitting position, then slowly curl back down. Arms should be at your sides for the whole exercise.

ACTIVE STRETCHING: Light, dynamic movements done with large ranges of motion to warm up joints and muscles. For example, you can lie on your back with your knees bent and both arms stretched out beside you. In a relaxed and gradual manner, let your knees fall to each side on the floor. Repeat approximately 5–10 times per side.

BACK EXTENSIONS: Performed lying on your stomach on the floor. Place both hands under your forehead with your elbows bent. Slowly lift your torso off the floor, and then lower it back down to the starting position. Always keep your neck straight and your eyes looking down at the floor.

BALL SQUATS: Similar to standing squats (see page 330), but this time you have a resistance ball behind your back. Place the ball against the wall and lean back into it. Your feet should be slightly wider than hip-width apart and about two feet from the wall. Lower to a squat with your knees bent to 90 degrees, and slowly return to the starting position.

BENT-KNEE PUSH-UPS: Similar to full push-ups, but your knees are on the ground. Your body should form a straight line from your shoulders to your knees. Slowly lower yourself down to the floor until your elbows reach a 90-degree angle; then push back up to the straight arm position and repeat.

BICEP CURLS: Stand with a weight in each hand, palms facing forward. Your knees should be straight but relaxed. Slowly lift the weights from straight arm position to fully bent position by curling your forearms up. Elbows will be bent and the weights will be near your shoulders at the final stage. Slowly lower the weights to the starting position; then repeat.

BIRD DOGS: Position yourself on your hands and knees on the floor. Keep your head in line with your spine and your lower back in a supported position, by slightly contracting your abdominal muscles. The goal of this exercise is to remain stable throughout your torso while moving your arms and legs. Slowly lift your left arm and reach it straight out in front of you. At the same time lift your right leg and stretch it in the opposite direction behind you. Hold for approximately two seconds, and then slowly lower your leg and arm to the starting position. Repeat with the right arm and left leg.

CALF RAISES: Stand on the edge of a stair with the front half of your foot on the step and the back half hanging over the step. Lower your heels down below the level of the stair's rise and then slowly raise yourself up to your toes.

CARDIO WARM-UP: Use a stationary bike at a low level of resistance. Choose the resistance level based on how much energy you have on a given day. You can also use a treadmill or go for a walk as a way of warming up.

DIPS: Sit on a bench or chair with your feet flat on the ground and your knees bent at 90 degrees. Move your feet about a foot farther away from the bench. Have your hands placed behind you on the edge of the bench, fingers facing forward. Slide your hips off the bench and then dip straight down so your hips are heading towards the floor. Once your elbows reach a 90-degree bend, push up to your starting position. Do as many reps as you can while maintaining good technique.

DOUBLE CURL-UPS: Lying on your back, cross your right leg over the left so the right ankle is resting on the left knee. Place your hands behind your head to support your neck. You are going to do a regular crunch with your upper body while at the same time lifting your left leg off the floor approximately one foot. Return both the upper and lower body to the floor starting position and repeat. Complete your repetitions on one side, and then switch your feet to repeat on the other side.

DUMBBELL CHEST PRESSES: Lie on your back on a bench with a weight in each hand. Start with arms extended straight up over your chest; then bend your arms as you slowly lower them down towards the bench until your elbows reach a 90-degree angle. Slowly return to straight arms and repeat. Make sure to keep breathing.

HAMSTRING CURLS: Lie on your back with both feet up on a resistance ball and your legs straight. Place your hands beside your hips. Slowly raise your hips off the mat. Only your shoulders and arms should be touching the mat at this time. Slowly bend your knees and curl the ball in towards you. Return to the straight-leg position and repeat.

HIP LIFTS: Lie on your back with your knees bent, both feet flat on the floor and your hands placed beside your hips. Slowly lift your hips and pelvis so that only your shoulders, arms and feet are touching the floor. Lower yourself back to the starting position and repeat. One-leg hip lifts are done in a similar manner. Instead of having two feet placed on the ground, you will have one foot straight in the air and one foot on the ground. From this position, slowly lift your hips and pelvis off the floor and return to the starting position to repeat.

LEG LIFTS (FRONT, SIDE AND BACK): This is a simple exercise that can be done anywhere. Using a wall or railing for balance, lift one leg straight to the front for the required repetitions (or until you get tired), then straight out to the side and then to the back. Make sure the movement is slow and controlled. You do not want your legs swinging back and forth. Finish the repetitions for one side; turn around and do the other side.

OBLIQUE TWISTS: Lie on your back, cross the right ankle over the left knee so that there is a space between your knees. Put your right arm behind your head, with the left arm straight out to the side. Lift your right shoulder towards the bent knee (you will be twisting on a diagonal across your abdomen). Slowly lower your torso back to the starting position and repeat. Finish all the repetitions on the right side; then switch legs and arms to do the left side.

ONE-ARM ROW: Using a bench or chair, place the right knee and the right hand on the bench. The weight will be in your left hand and your left foot will be on the floor beside the bench. Make sure your back is in a straight position and your abdominals are slightly contracted to support your lower back. Let your left arm hang straight down from the shoulder. This is your starting position. From there, bend your left elbow and lift the weight up towards your side. When you reach the side of your body, slowly lower the weight down and repeat for the required number on that side. When you are finished, turn 180 degrees with your left knee and hand on the bench and place the weight in your right hand to repeat on that side.

PNF STRETCHING: PNF stands for "Proprioceptive Neuromuscular Facilitation." This kind of stretching is done with a partner or therapist who stretches you while you are trying to relax and contract muscles. This is an ideal way to work on your flexibility during a time when you have little energy to stretch by yourself. If you can work with someone who is trained in this form of stretching, it is recommended. If not, stretching on your own is equally important to your overall routine, so leave time at the end of each workout for a stretch.

REVERSE ABDOMINAL LIFTS: Lie on your back with both feet straight in the air. Reach both toes straight to the ceiling so that your hips come slightly off the floor. Slowly lower your hips to the starting position and repeat.

STANDING SQUATS: Stand with your legs slightly wider than shoulder-width apart, and squat down as if you were going to sit in a chair. Once your knees are bent to a 90-degree angle, return to the starting position and repeat.

STEP-UPS: With weights in each hand, place one foot on the first step of a set of stairs. (Use the second step if you feel comfortable doing so.) Keep this foot on the step for all of the repetitions. Simply step up onto the stair with the other foot and then step down again. Finish all the reps on one side; then repeat on the other side.

STRAIGHT-LEG STRETCH: This is based on a Pilates exercise and it is a great core stabilizer. Lying on your back, with both legs straight in the air, contract your abdominals, slowly lower one leg down to the floor, and then return it to the starting position. Keep the lifted leg as straight as possible throughout the movement. Repeat the stretch with the other leg. Your back should not move during this exercise. To do this exercise properly you must have enough strength in your abdominals to maintain a stable position in your lower back. If you find your back is arching off the floor, this exercise is too advanced for your abdominal strength and it is best to substitute another abdominal exercise.

SWIMMERS: Lie on your stomach with your arms straight out in front of you and your legs straight. Your forehead should be resting on the floor. Lift one leg at a time as if you were doing a flutter kick in swimming, and at the same time lift the opposite arm. Repeat on the other side, alternating until you are done.

TRICEP EXTENSIONS: Stand next to a bench and rest one knee on the bench. Lean over and support your upper-body weight by resting one hand on the bench. Hold a weight in the hand that is hanging by your side. Bend that arm to 90 degrees, keeping your elbow close to your body. From the bent elbow position, slowly straighten the arm with the weight. Return to the starting position and repeat.

Dr. Stacy Irvine is a Chiropractor and Personal Trainer in Toronto, Ontario. She's also one of Canada's top female fitness experts, appearing on Balance Television *and* E-Talk Daily.

Glossary

Adriamycin: trade name for doxorubicin, a chemotherapy drug nicknamed the "red devil"

anastrozole: see *Arimidex*

ankylosing spondylitis: a progressive disease of the spinal column that leads to mobility loss

anterior: in medical usage, at or towards the front of the body

areola: the pigmented area of skin surrounding the nipple

Arimidex: trade name for anastrozole, an aromatase inhibitor

aromatase inhibitors: medications that stop conversion of peripheral hormones to estrogen in the bloodstream

Ativan: trade name for lorazepam, a tranquilizer

atypia: the state of cells that appear abnormal when viewed under a microscope

biopsy: a small sample of tissue removed for microscopic examination in order to discover the cause or nature of a disease. In a core, or needle, biopsy, the tissue is removed through a hollow needle. A stereotactic core biopsy uses x-ray images and a computer guidance system to accurately pinpoint the biopsy site. A punch biopsy is a skin biopsy done by using a small, sharp tool that looks like a cookie-cutter to remove a circular piece of skin.

BRCA1/BRCA2: hereditary gene mutations associated with breast and ovarian cancers

breast-conserving surgery: removal of a tumour without removing the entire breast; see also *lumpectomy*

broad-spectrum: widely effective; usually used in reference to antibiotics

calcifications: deposits of calcium salts in body tissues

carcinoma: a cancer of a surface layer of the body

cellulitis: infection of the skin

chemotherapy: the use of drugs to attack cancer cells and stop their growth

Colace: trade name for docusate sodium, a stool softener; used to treat constipation

cortisone: a steroid often used to treat allergic skin reactions

cystoscopy: examination of the inside of the bladder using a scope with a camera and light attached

Cytoxan: trade name for cyclophosphamide, a chemotherapy drug; among its many harmful side effects is a decrease in blood formation by the bone marrow.

dermatitis, contact: inflammation of the skin caused by contact with an irritant; causes redness, swelling, blisters and itching, among other symptoms.

dexamethasone: a synthetic steroid drug used to counteract the side effects of chemotherapy, for example, nausea

Dilaudid: trade name for hydromorphone hydrochloride, a morphine substitute used as a painkiller

domperidone: a drug used to control nausea and vomiting

dose-dense: a term used to describe chemotherapy in which higher doses are given at shorter intervals

doxorubicin: see *Adriamycin*

ductal carcinoma: breast cancer that begins in the walls of the milk ducts

endorphins: substances produced by the body that provide relief of pain and stress

Eprex: trade name for a synthetic form of epoetin alfa; used to counteract low hemoglobin levels in patients undergoing chemotherapy

estrogen-positive: describes a cancer that has receptors on its cells that are stimulated by estrogen, causing further growth. Approximately 70% of breast cancers are estrogen-positive; most of these are found in older women.

fibrous breast lumps: non-cancerous solid lumps composed of fibrous tissue

filgrastim: see *Neupogen*

gadolinium: an element, also known as gadodiamide, used in MRIs to provide contrast between normal and abnormal tissue. After it is injected into a vein it accumulates in the abnormal tissue, causing those areas to appear brighter on the MRI.

gastritis, erosive: inflammation of the stomach that causes minor damage to the stomach lining, often with some bleeding

G-CSF: granulocyte colony-stimulating factor, a growth factor that helps stimulate production of white blood cells, which fight infection

genetic counseling: the testing of parents to determine whether their children are likely to suffer from genetic disorders or conditions associated with certain gene mutations

goserelin acetate: see *Zoladex*

grade: a measure of a tumour's severity, based on how abnormal the cancer cells look under a microscope and how quickly the tumour is likely to grow and spread. Each type of cancer has its own grading system.

granulocytes: a class of white blood cells that includes neutrophils, among other types

hematoma: an accumulation of partially clotted blood within the body

hemoglobin: the iron-containing protein in red blood cells; low hemoglobin leads to anemia

heparin: a substance used to prevent blood from clotting

Herceptin: trade name for trastuzumab, a type of monoclonal antibody, which is a laboratory-produced substance that can locate and bind to cancer cells. It blocks the effects of a protein that sends growth signals to breast cancer cells.

hormonal therapy: treatment used to slow or stop the growth of breast and other cancers by giving synthetic hormones or other drugs to block the body's natural hormones.

hydromorphone hydrochloride: see *Dilaudid*

hysterosalpingogram: an x-ray examination of the uterus, fallopian tubes and ovaries using contrast medium to detect blockages and abnormalities

immune system: the lymphatic system; the body's defences against invasion by microbes, cancer cells or foreign tissues

immuno-suppression: a state in which the immune system is prevented from attacking infection or foreign bodies

in situ: Latin for "in place"; used to refer to early cancers that have not spread to surrounding tissues

interval cancer: breast cancer that occurs within three years of a
negative screening test (such as a mammogram)

intra-abdominal: occurring within the abdominal cavity

intravenous line: a fine tube inserted into a vein; used to introduce
medication directly into the blood system

invasion: when cancer spreads beyond the tissue in which it developed,
growing into surrounding healthy tissues; see also *lymphovascular
invasion; micro-invasion*

labia minora: Latin for "small lips"; the inner parts of the external
female genitals that form the entrance to the vagina and urethra

lesion: an injury, wound, infection or any other kind of abnormality in
the body

lobular carcinoma: breast cancer that begins in the lobules, or milk-
producing glands

localization: determining and marking the location of a disease area.
Needle localization uses very thin needles or guide-wires to mark
the location of an abnormal area of tissue so that it can be surgically
removed. MRI or x-ray is used to guide the wire to the correct
location and a collapsible hook at the end of the needle keeps it in
place until the surgery is done.

lorazepam: see *Ativan*

lumpectomy: surgery to remove a tumour and a small amount of normal
tissue (margins) around it; see also *breast-conserving surgery*

lymphedema: swelling of the tissues caused by blocked or missing lymph
channels

lymph nodes: small, bean-shaped bodies found in groups in the armpits,
groin, neck and other parts of the body. Part of the immune system,
they produce antibodies, but can also cause the spread of cancer. See
also *sentinel node*

lymphovascular invasion: when cancer cells invade the blood vessels
or lymphatic channels of the tumour, increasing the possibility
of spread to the lymph nodes or other areas in the body; see also
lymphovascular invasion; micro-invasion

mammogram: examination of the breasts with low-radiation x-rays to
detect changes in density that might indicate breast cancer

mammographic sensitivity: the percentage of tumours detected by
mammogram

margin: the edge or border of normal tissue removed in cancer surgery

mastectomy: surgical removal of the breast. A bilateral mastectomy removes both breasts. A skin-sparing mastectomy takes only the skin that must be removed to prevent further spread of cancer (nipple, areola and biopsy incision area); the remaining pouch of skin can be used for reconstruction or an implant.

menopause: the cessation of menstruation and reproductive capability that occurs naturally in women around the average age of 50; may be induced earlier by surgical removal of the reproductive organs, chemotherapy or radiation to the pelvic area

metastasis: the spread of cancer to another part of the body from the site where it originally developed, usually through the bloodstream or lymphatic system. The new sites of disease are called metastases.

methylene blue: a dye used to stain certain parts of the body before or during surgery

micro-invasion: in ductal carcinoma in situ, when a small number of cancer cells partly break through the duct wall. Undetectable on a mammogram, it is usually found by the pathologist examining tissue from a biopsy under a microscope, but is easy to miss when the area of invasion is very small compared to the piece of breast tissue; see also *invasion; lymphovascular invasion*

motility agent: a medication used to reduce constipation

MRI: magnetic resonance imaging, a scanning technique that uses strong electromagnets in conjunction with radio waves to detect abnormalities in body tissues

needle localization: see *localization*

Neupogen: trade name for filgrastim, a protein that stimulates the production of white blood cells to decrease the risk of infection

neutropenia: an abnormally low number of neutrophils in the blood, increasing the risk of infection

neutrophils: white blood cells that help the body fight bacteria and fungi, heal wounds and help protect the body against foreign matter

Nexium: trade name for esomeprazole, a drug used to counteract excess stomach acid

oncologist: a doctor who specializes in the treatment of cancer. A medical oncologist specializes in cancer treatment with chemotherapy, and a radiation oncologist specializes in radiation treatments.

ondansetron: a drug used to prevent nausea and vomiting

osteopenia: a condition of low bone density not severe enough to be classed as osteoporosis

osteoporosis: a condition of fragile, porous bones caused by loss of protein and mineral content

paclitaxel: see *Taxol*

pathology: a branch of medical science that deals with disease processes, causes and effects on the body; also used to refer to the results of pathological investigations

pectoral muscles: muscles of the upper chest that control the shoulder blade and some arm movements. In reconstructive surgery, implants are placed underneath the pectoral muscles, against the ribs.

portacath: a device inserted in the upper chest wall between the collarbone and breast to make drawing blood and receiving chemotherapy easier and more comfortable. The port is about the size of a thick quarter, and insertion and removal are simple procedures using local anesthetic. It allows medication to be introduced directly into the main blood supply to the heart so that it can be delivered quickly to all parts of the body.

prednisone: a synthetic steroid drug used to relieve inflammation

Procytox: see *Cytoxan*

prosthesis: an artificial body part used to replace one that has been lost through accident or disease

proton pump inhibitors: drugs used to reduce excess acid in the stomach

push: a method of intravenous drug administration in which the fluid is slowly pushed in rather than simply being allowed to drip

radiation therapy: the use of ionizing radiation (e.g., x-rays) and radioactive isotopes to treat cancerous tumours

ranitidine: a drug used to treat heartburn and excess stomach acidity

receptors: see *estrogen-positive*

reconstruction: surgery to rebuild a body part removed or damaged because of accident or disease. Breast reconstruction can be done by using tissue from the abdomen (TRAM) or by inserting synthetic implants.

recurrence: the reappearance of cancer after treatment. Most breast cancer recurrences happen in the first three to five years after initial treatment, either locally (in the treated breast or near the mastectomy scar) or somewhere else in the body (most commonly the lymph nodes, bones, liver or lungs).

saline: a salt-and-water solution that matches the salt content of body fluids; used intravenously for maintaining healthy fluid levels

sentinel node: the first lymph node that receives lymphatic drainage from a tumour

serratus anterior: a muscle anchored to the sides of the ribs that works with the pectoral muscle to move the shoulder blade

subclavian vein: the main vein that transports blood from the arms to the lungs

TAHBSO: total abdominal hysterectomy and bilateral salpingo-oophorectomy, or removal of the uterus and both ovaries and fallopian tubes

tamoxifen: a drug that blocks estrogen receptors; used in the treatment of breast cancer

Taxol: trade name for paclitaxel, a drug that slows or stops the growth of cancer cells

topical: in medical usage, something that affects or is applied to the outside of the body (i.e., the skin or hair)

TRAM: the transverse *rectus abdominis* muscle, located in the lower abdomen between the waist and the pubic bone. Tissue from this area is used for a TRAM flap reconstruction after mastectomy.

transference: a psychological phenomenon in which feelings about one person or thing are transferred to another, often unrelated person or thing.

ultrasound: a medical imaging method that uses sound waves to examine internal organs and soft tissues. Targeted ultrasound uses a higher level of resolution to achieve more detailed information. Ultrasound is also used to treat painful inflammations.

Zoladex: trade name for goserelin acetate, a drug used to stop the production of estrogen in the body

Index

Gabereau, Vicki, 47, 207, 208, 242, 272
gadolinium, 35
gastric irritation, 128, 145
G-CSF (granulocyte colony-stimulating
      factor), 112
Gemini Awards, 103, 163
gene mutations, 57–58, 178, 229
genetic testing, 14, 57–58, 88
Glina, Cherie, 263, 276, 278
Globe and Mail (M's column in),
      129–34, 186–90, 248–49
Good Morning America, 25–26
Gore, Tipper, 21
goserelin acetate. *See* Zoladex
Grace (housekeeper), 143, 144, 145,
      282
granulocytes. *See* white blood cells
grief, 17–18
Gupta, Sanjay, 25

hair loss, 111, 130, 135–37, 143. *See
      also* wigs
   baldness, 143–44, 145–46
   baldness in public, 162–67, 208,
      216, 272–73, 299
   caps and hats, 161, 294
   children's reaction to, 97, 106,
      145, 161, 170, 271–73, 293–94,
      298–99
   eyebrows, lashes and nostril hair,
      144–45, 191
   and identity, 161–62
   regrowth, 277, 290, 300
   styling during, 135–36
Haliskie, Brent, 243
Health Canada, 21
heart disease, 50
hematoma, 232
hemoglobin, 166–67, 168
Henderson, Gordon, 242–43
heparin, 126–27
Herceptin, 90

Hershkop, Marlon, 63–64
Her-s/neu protein, 90
Holmes, Robert, 243
hormones, precursor, 197. *See also*
      estrogen
Houston International Film Festival,
      252
humour, 82, 83, 153–54, 216
   as helpful, 152–59, 214–15,
      235, 291–92
Hurst, Robert, 77–78, 99–100
hysterectomy, 178, 201, 229–33
hysterosalpingogram, 20

identity, 102, 161–62, 170
implants, 102, 154, 228, 245–46
   expanders for, 102, 210, 221–23,
      225–28, 234, 236
infection, 75, 110–11, 123, 208, 246,
      290
insomnia
   after surgery, 69, 277
   from grief, 18
   from medications, 115, 128, 129
   medications for, 145
   menopause-induced, 184, 233
Internet chat, 44
invasion, 49, 87–88, 89–90
   lymphovascular, 175, 177
   micro-invasion, 32, 81
isolation, 169. *See also* privacy
   feelings of, 79–80, 242
   need for, 109, 112–13, 148

Janice (patient), 160–61
Jason (son), 4, 14–18, 52, 245
   death of, 14, 17, 148, 259, 267,
      279, 306
Jeanette (Lawrence's wife), 181, 182
Jenna (daughter), 259–79
   and Amanda, 268
   birthday, 164–65

343

and M's surgeries, 70, 80, 232
reactions to M's cancer, 80, 83, 121,
    196, 298, 300–301
support from, 170–71
McCready, David, 27–28, 29, 239
and lumpectomy, 38–41, 54, 62–63,
    66–67, 75–76, 138–39
and mastectomies, 197–98, 200, 221
and pathology report, 81, 86, 97
and post-surgery complications,
    73–74, 75
McGraw, Phil ("Dr. Phil"), 25, 141
medications. *See also specific medications*
allergies to, 68, 111, 168, 211
anti-nausea, 110, 128, 169
costs of, 110, 112, 145, 212
for pain, 274–75, 276–77
reactions to, 275, 277–78
schedule for, 170, 299
melanoma, 239
menopause, 226
chemically induced, 175, 226, 229
estrogen production after, 178
surgical, 197, 229, 230
symptoms of, 184, 226, 233
Meschino, Wendy, 58
Mesley, Wendy, 185, 186
metastases, 49, 52–53
morphine, 68, 211
Morris, Scott, 22, 23
mortality, 95
mouth sores, 128, 145
MRI (magnetic resonance imaging),
    30, 32–33
of breasts, 33–36, 42, 46–47, 56–57,
    175
localization with, 46–47, 53, 59–60,
    76, 175
monitoring with, 87, 139
progressive phase, 35, 53
results, 37, 46–47
Murphy, Joan, 178–79, 229, 232, 233

Murray (friend), 171–72
muscles, pectoral, 102, 227, 236, 246

National Breast Cancer Awareness
    Month, 251
National Cancer Institute (U.S.), 92
nausea
from chemotherapy, 113, 118, 145,
    164
remedies for, 110, 128, 169
needle localization, 57
Neulasta (pegfilgrastim), 212
Neupogen (filgrastim), 96, 112, 118,
    123
neutropenia, 112
neutrophils. *See* white blood cells
Nexium, 145
90th Parallel, 242
nipple (reconstruction), 102, 238–39
North American Menopause Society, 252
nuclear tracers, 63–64, 79

ondansetron, 110, 121, 128
On Death and Dying (Kübler-Ross), 36
O'Reagan, Seamus, 100, 130–31
osteopenia, 202
osteoporosis, 128
Osteoporosis Society of Canada, 163
ovarian cancer, 57–58, 141, 229
ovaries, 178, 229. *See also* hysterectomy

paclitaxel. *See* Taxol
pain
after surgery, 69, 221–22, 225,
    230–31, 246
medication for, 274–75, 276–77
from torn muscle, 227
Paszt, Brent, 100
pathology
reports on, 40, 81–82, 86–87, 88–90
second opinion on, 91–92, 95, 101
specimens for, 66–67, 79